Caring & Cooking for the Allergic Child

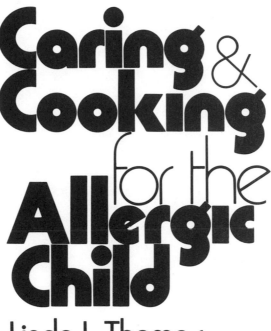

Caring & Cooking for the Allergic Child

Linda L. Thomas

Foreword by Allen Sosin, M.D., F.A.A.P.
Introduction by Katharine Crossman, M.S.,
Registered Dietician

Revised Edition

Sterling Publishing Co., Inc.   New York
Oak Tree Press Co., Ltd London & Sydney

Published in 1980 by
Sterling Publishing Co., Inc.
Two Park Avenue
New York, N.Y. 10016

Distributed in the United Kingdom and Australia by Oak Tree Press Co., Ltd.

ISBN 0-8069-5552-X
Previously
ISBN 0-87749-593-9
Oak Tree 7061-2687-4

Printed in U.S.A.

Library of Congress Catalog Card No.: 79-91379

Contents

CHAPTER 1.

CHAPTER 2.

CHAPTER 3.

CHAPTER 4.

CHAPTER 5.

CHAPTER 6.

FOR DAVID

Foreword

Allergy is a chronic ailment that is manifested by a hypersensitive reaction in your body. This can range in severity from irritating to debilitating. It is so common that most families are directly or indirectly affected by it. Fortunately, most are only inconvenienced by it. The symptoms are dependent on which organ of the body has the reaction, and can vary even in the same individual. Of course, when a hypersensitive reaction occurs, we suffer from a loss of time, money, and comfort.

The treatment of allergy is very difficult because of the complexity of causes. We are allergic to many factors that work in combination to produce symptoms. We each have a threshold, above which we have symptoms and below which we are free of them. Therefore we might not show signs of allergy with each exposure or in the same way alleviate the symptoms each time we withdraw the causative material. This, of course, makes the determination of cause much more difficult and requires that the patient and/or parent be a first-class detective, trying to track down and to remove causes.

Eliminating these causal factors is not always possible. Frequently we try too hard and make the "cure" worse than the "disease." Unfortunately there is no true "cure" for allergies. In the last twenty-five years our scientific knowledge has grown remarkably; however, the basic treatment is still to remove the cause and treat symptomatically. It is not reasonable to expect that the patient live in a glass cage, free of causal factors. Often we can eliminate or markedly reduce symptoms with control of environment and/or diet. Even patients on a hyposensitization routine require control of causative factors.

The control of diet can be simple, such as removal of strawberries, or extremely difficult, when it is extensive. I find most resistance in parents and children to strict dietary controls, and I have developed the greatest empathy for these problems. It is indeed difficult to plan balanced, nutritious, appetizing meals and snacks for any family, but to complicate it with restricted foods, problem additives, and poor labeling, requires a wizard with unlimited patience.

Mrs. Thomas has had to live with the formidable task and has done a remarkable job with her own son. As a pediatric allergist I am grateful that she has had the ability. to create this book and to offer it as an aid for other parents. Nobody can pull all the answers into one volume. You must individualize your treatment and use this and other sources to make your life and that of your child as normal as it is possible.

Allen Sosin, M.D., F.A.A.P.

XI

Preface

There is nothing so sad as a child who gets violently ill from apparently everything he eats—unless it is the frustrated parent who doesn't know how to help him!

When you were told that your child had malabsorption syndrome and/or several food allergies, you believed there would be only minor adjustments to your cooking routine. You started reading food labels and found that many favorite brands contained at least one ingredient not allowed in your child's diet. Then you decided to cook from scratch. But most of your recipes contained eggs or flour and you didn't know how to eliminate them from the recipe. Perhaps you started reading at the library. You found there are many recipe books but there were few recipes in them that didn't include at least one ingredient that must be eliminated from your child's diet.

Now you really begin to panic! Your mind swims with questions:

1. What do I feed my baby when he can't eat many of the prepared foods?

2. What can I feed a toddler on a gluten-free diet to replace the finger foods other babies enjoy?

3. What can I give my child to eat at his birthday party that won't make him feel different than his playmates?

4. How can he enjoy Halloween and other treat times when all the candy contains corn products?

5. How do I keep him from becoming bored and rebelling at the restrictions of his diet?

6. Who can stand rice cereal at every breakfast? Isn't there some way to add taste variety to it?

7. How can I cook for my allergic child without cooking a second meal for the rest of the family?

If these questions have gone through your mind this book will provide the answers and hopefully help calm your fears.

Brand names will be used in recipes where they are required, not as an endorsement of the product, but as an aid to you in preparing the food. At the end of the book is a list of food brands and products that have been found helpful. Be sure to reread the labels often, however, as ingredients are often changed with improvements in the product.

Above all, don't despair. You will discover, as I have, that cooking for the allergic child can be a challenge and a satisfaction with the reward a happier, more contented, healthier child.

L.L.T.
South Lyon, Michigan
August 1973

Acknowledgments

Without the assistance of so many wonderful people this book would never have been written. My deepest appreciation goes to my family, who lived through the trial and error of innumerable recipes since the conception of this diet; to Dr. Allen Sosin and Dr. Max Garber who encouraged me to write the book and waded through the manuscript to make corrections; to Kathy Crossman who reassured me when I felt I was starving my baby and who has been a tremendous help with the research for this book (I had some very difficult questions for her!). I treasure her friendship. To the Oakland County, Michigan, Health Department for the help they offered, especially Mary Massini, our school health nurse, for steering me to the right people; to the librarians at the South Lyon Public Library who always kept an eye out for books and articles that might help in my research; to the University of Michigan Medical Library for their vast supply of information; to Norma Lambert who helped correct my manuscript; to my sister-in-law, Barbara Havershaw, for contributing recipes and her typing expertise; and to my dear friend, Joan Unger, whose help and encouragement with my writing efforts mean more to me than she will ever know.

The Dietician as a Resource Person for the Parent of an Allergic Child

Since the planning of foods to be included on an allergic child's diet often involves gathering much detailed information about the composition and ingredients in food products, the dietitian can be a definite help to the parents in obtaining this information. She is part of the professional medical team, knows not only the chemistry of foods, but also how the body breaks down food and either uses or reacts to it. She can help to interpret the medical information from the physician and translate it into the language of the diet.

The dietitian also has a depth of knowledge of nutrition not often possessed by physicians and can evaluate the child's diet for nutritional value and recommend changes to the physician if needed.

The dietitian will usually have the following resources available:

1. Lists of foods which do and do not contain the allergen.
2. Addresses for obtaining further information about specific food products.
3. Knowledge of various methods of food preparation.
4. Food composition books with which to evaluate the nutritional adequacy of the diet.

Dietitians are most commonly found in local hospitals, but are becoming more available in local health departments. If a dietitian is not available to you, ask the local hospital for the name of the president of the local or state dietetic association. She should be able to refer you to a dietitian close to you.

Allergy diets of such complexity as that described here by Mrs. Thomas are not encountered very often by dietitians. Therefore, the dietitians may have to gather materials continuously as more and more is discovered about the child's allergy. For example, David drinks diluted soybean milk, which is a legume, but is in general, allergic to the botanical family of legumes. In our search for an answer why carob powder could not be used, we began to look at botanical relationships and discovered that carob is a member of the legume family.

The list which is presented in this book is invaluable in guessing whether or not, if the child is allergic to one food in a given group he might also be allergic to other foods in the same group.

Mrs. Thomas's ability to devise delicious recipes to make food an enjoyable experience for David will be a stimulus to parents of other allergic children who turn to this book for help.

Katharine Crossman, M.S.
Registered Dietitian

How to Use This Book for Maximum Benefit

1. Learn through work with your allergist what foods your child can and cannot tolerate. Keep a list of these foods taped to the inside of your cupboard door for quick reference. Soon you will have the list memorized and won't need it as often, but keep it there anyway for the use of others who may come in to care for your child. It is essential that you keep the list current by adding any newly tried foods.
2. Read through the recipes in this book to find those that are usable for your child. If a recipe seems unsuitable for your needs, read it again, considering each ingredient carefully. Possibly one spice could be substituted for another, or left out, or one gluten-free flour exchanged for another.
3. Compare the recipe with others having similar ingredients for substitution ideas.
4. Before changing recipes, read the substitution charts carefully and realize that some experimentation and a few failures are probably inevitable, but you will develop ease and have success in adapting recipes for your child. Think of it as a detective game.
5. If you are new to cooking with special flour, use these recipes until you are used to the flavors and textures available. Be sure to taste the foods yourself so you will understand your child's likes and dislikes. You may be surprised to find that you enjoy some of the foods yourself.
6. Go through your family's favorite recipes and see if they can be adapted to this style of cooking. Possibly rice flour could be substituted for wheat flower, or meat breaded with crushed allowable cereal. Your imagination is given free rein when formulating recipes for an allergy. Don't be afraid to try!
7. Don't make double batches of recipes, since dough often becomes heavy in large amounts.

1

Coping With the Allergic Child

"I'm afraid to take my eyes off of this child. He's always eating something he shouldn't have!" How many times I expressed that thought! At times I think fear for my child's safety was all that kept me going. I lost five pounds trying to keep up with my two-year-old. He was always eating what his sisters ate, not realizing the food could harm him. He ran constantly, never walked anywhere. I soon learned that some allergic or celiac children are hyperactive just because their digestive system is constantly uncomfortable. This keeps them keyed up all the time. They don't sleep well at night, they are often wakeful and restless. It is comforting to know that when their diet is regulated and they start to feel better they settle down.

It is easy to regulate the diet of an infant because his diet is very limited to begin with. If one formula bothers him, perhaps another will work well. You simply add foods slowly, one at a time, from his formula on. Your pediatrician will help you to formulate a proper diet. A toddler or older child is much more difficult to regulate because he already has favorite foods and a more varied diet. It is very important that you follow your doctor's instructions and work closely with him. You will have difficulty with your child sneaking foods for awhile but eventually even a toddler will learn to say, "No, that gives me a tummy ache."

To accomplish this you will have to be a tyrant for a time and faithfully restrict your toddler. He will find it difficult to understand why he could eat cookies yesterday but he can't eat them today. He will take food and find a place to hide while he eats it, or lie on top of it protectively like a football player on a ball.

But when you start making him his own desserts and exchanging the no-no for *his* cookies, he soon starts sneaking *his* cookies and loses interest in the wheat-flour type. Soon he loses his taste for milk, eggs, wheat or corn; if indeed he ever had a taste for them. Often a child will not accept a food that he is allergic to, even before the allergy has been diagnosed. You may find, however, that your child sneaks the forbidden food at intervals just to see if it still bothers him. When he does get sick from the food be sure to tell him, without becoming angry, what the offender was. This teaches him more effectively than any scolding, why he must refuse certain foods when they are offered to him by others. Remember that some children become ill from the cooking odor of eggs, tomatoes or corn. Watch your children for such a reaction.

Before your child was diagnosed you probably felt like an overprotective parent. You seemed to meet yourself coming and going at the doctor's office. The receptionist began to recognize your voice over the phone before you could identify yourself. You wondered if you were turning your child into a hypochondriac. Believe me, once his diet becomes regulated you won't have to see your doctor so often with colds, tummy aches, sore throats, bronchitis, and the like. Allergic children whose diets are uncontrolled seem to be more susceptible to illness than other children, perhaps because they are run-down all the time.

Having your child officially diagnosed as allergic or as suffering from malabsorption syndrome is one thing. The acceptance of the diagnosis by one or both parents is yet another. Mother often feels that the problem was somehow caused by her while she was pregnant. Father feels that there must be something wrong with him that his child is not healthy and "normal." Many a father will not accept the fact that his child has a chronic illness.

My husband, although allergic himself, felt that I was being too fussy in the preparation of our son's food and that I was causing the problems myself. To him, the boy seemed fine; but that was because his diet was already regulated. Even after many discussions about this he gave him ice cream, cookies, soda pop, Jell-O, etc. and the child was fine perhaps for a week. Then it took three weeks to control his diarrhea. My husband now realizes that there is a real problem, but if we all cooperate the problem may be brought under reasonable control.

You will undoubtedly have similar problems with relatives and neighbors. Let them know that the child is your responsibility; you have to live with him and you would rather live with him well than sick.

Ask neighbors not to feed him anything that you have not approved. When visiting, take his food to supplement what your hostesss may have prepared for dinner; and stick to his diet no matter what the other people say. But do be diplomatic. If you have problems with some doting relative sitting by your child and sneaking food to him, place the child between you and your husband next time. People will soon realize that you mean what you say. And they will soon notice the difference in the child's looks and actions if they are around him much. Remember not to talk about your child when he is listening or he may begin to feel that he is abnormal. The limitations imposed on an allergic child will often create a feeling of self-pity. A parental attitude of encouragement may determine whether he becomes an emotional invalid or a self-assured, self-sufficient person, who takes responsibility for his own diet and avoidance measures. Occasional self-pity is to be expected, but not dwelled upon. The child should learn that every person has imperfections that he must learn to live with (wearing glasses, corrective shoes, mouth braces, etc.). How he copes with his imperfection shows strength of character.

He has more rules than most children just because he is so restricted in what he can eat. Don't worry about making him hang up his clothes or pick up his toys. Encourage these things, certainly, and help him, but don't punish him if he doesn't do them on his own initiative. You will have a much more cooperative child to live with and encounter much less rebellion against those rules that are the most necessary.

Most important is a good basic understanding of his allergic problem. The answers to many of your questions along this line will be found in the next chapter.

2

What Makes Him Tick?

WHAT ARE ALLERGIES? Allergies are an inherited condition which is passed to the infant by his parents. If one parent is allergic and the other is not, there is a chance that half your children will be allergic. An allergic mother transmits allergy to her child twice as frequently as an allergic father. If both parents are allergic, the probability of having an allergic child rises to three out of four. These children often develop allergy at an earlier age than the child with one allergic parent. Occasionally a child shows up with allergy when there is no family history of allergies, but this is only a small percentage of the total allergic children.

National Health Organizations estimate that: approximately 31 million individuals, or 15 per cent of the U.S. population, suffer from some form of allergy; 12 per cent of Americans are allergic to food additives; milk allergy is more frequent in boys than girls; and, 40 per cent of milk-sensitive infants develop gluten sensitivity. Those with the most severe gastrointestinal reactions as babies tend to replace them with respiratory allergies later in life. There are some measures that the mother can take during her pregnancy to help prevent early and severe allergies in her young infant. While this information has come too late to help with the allergic child you now have, it may be of benefit to you in a later pregnancy.

1. If the mother is allergic herself, she should avoid any food to which she is allergic or foods that cause her to experience the discomfort of heartburn, gas, nausea, etc.

2. Don't eat any food in excess even if you do feel that it is good for you.

3. Since milk and eggs are the major causes of gastrointestinal allergy in infants, it is wise to eliminate large amounts of either. Egg or milk cooked in food won't cause much of a problem unless proportionately high in total content—such as egg salad, cheese, custard puddings, angel food cake, instant breakfast drinks, etc. One pint of milk per day, plus prenatal vitamins, will give you a sufficient amount of calcium and phosphorus.

4. Every effort should be made to breastfeed your newborn because many allergies are caused by cow's milk formulas. While you are nursing it is important to

continue to follow the guidelines for eating during pregnancy since the food you eat goes into your milk.

ALLERGIC REACTIONS. Allergy diets are very tricky. After you have followed one faithfully for six months or so you may find yourself becoming lax and surprisingly, Johnny doesn't have a reaction to that extra slice of bread as he did before you started his diet. He's not allergic any more! Until the next week, when he has a severe reaction. This may seem confusing to you unless your allergist has explained to you that each allergic person has an individual threshold of tolerance. This chart may help to explain how an allergic reaction occurs.

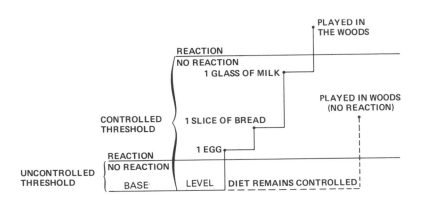

Before your child began diet control his threshold was at the uncontrolled threshold line. Perhaps he could eat one slice of bread and not become very ill, but give him a sandwich with two slices and watch out! After a trip to the allergist and tests to determine just what he is allergic to, the doctor gave you a list of foods to eliminate from his diet. If you followed the instructions carefully, you were able to raise his threshold to the controlled level. As long as you keep his diet controlled he can tolerate much better the things in his environment that give him difficulty.

Once his diet is controlled and his threshold raised, you will discover that he can tolerate the occasional lollipop that Aunt Jenny slips him without getting into difficulty. (A word of warning here, however. A toddler cannot understand why he can have a lollipop today and not tomorrow. It is best to insist there be *NO* exceptions to the rules until he is old enough to be reasoned with.)

If there is a food that causes severe reactions, don't even be tempted to try it without your doctor's instructions. One try may raise your child above this threshold if the food given is one to which he is highly allergic. The ideal situation is to stay away from the problem foods completely and to keep his tolerance threshold at the very highest possible level, but this is next to impossible with a child. You will simply have to be content with doing the best you can and hope that any reactions will be mild ones. The most common symptoms of food allergy are:

DIGESTIVE

Nausea
Vomiting
Cramps-Colic
Bloating
Indigestion
Diarrhea
Constipation

SKIN

Itch
Rash
Hives
Eczema
Canker Sores
Swollen Lips,
    Tongue, Mouth

RESPIRATORY

Runny Nose
Sneezing
Cough
Wheeze
Hoarseness
Sinus Infection
Earaches
Dizziness

SYSTEMIC

Muscular Ache
Swollen Glands
    (especially neck)
Low-Grade Fever
Shock
Pallor

NEUROLOGIC

Headache & Migraine
Altered Activity
Altered Behavior
Chilliness
Nervous Tension

To counteract these effects of allergy, a diet must be followed faithfully, eliminating the guilty foods.

USING THIS DIET FOR CELIAC DISEASE. Malabsorption is basically the inability of the small intestine to absorb certain nutrients—proteins, fats or sugars. Any food that is not absorbed correctly is eliminated from the body without the removal of vitamins and other essential nutrients. The child with uncontrolled malabsorption is a very sickly child. He is not growing normally; he has abnormal stools more often than not; he doesn't sleep well because of intestinal cramps; his abdomen is bloated and he is often tired and cranky. There are three basic types of malabsorption syndrome.

1. *Cystic Fibrosis*—This is inherited. The actual cause remains unknown, but many of the symptoms are the result of extremely thick mucus which blocks ducts in the lungs and pancreas. This disease is not to be confused with ordinary diarrhea. In cystic fibrosis the stools are foul-smelling and show undigested food with a thick mucous covering. Because the ability to absorb fats is impaired, the disease requires a diet to control fat intake plus supplementary enzymes to increase absorption. Consequently cystic fibrosis requires an entirely different treatment than the diet in this book.

2. *Sugar Intolerance*—This is not the same as diabetes because some carbo-

hydrates can be utilized. The main difficulty is the inability to digest milk and cane sugars. These are complex sugars, and the sugar-splitting enzyme that is necessary to break them down so that the body can use them, is missing. As a result the sugars are eliminated through the bowels, causing diarrhea.

This is quite rare, but sometimes a false impression of sugar intolerance can be given to the doctor because of an extremely high sugar intake in the diet. For this reason it is a good idea to add as little sugar to the recipes as your child will accept, and not necessarily as much as the recipe calls for. Brown sugar is about twice as sweet as white sugar, and therefore could be used in smaller amounts. Honey is easier to digest because it is high in simple sugar, and this may be all that is needed to solve a suspected case of sugar intolerance.

3. *Celiac Disease*— This condition can be controlled with the diet in this book because gluten, the culprit, has been eliminated from all recipes. Celiac disease is actually improperly named because it is in reality not a disease but a body condition caused by a deficiency of the enzyme which is needed to break down the gluten in wheat and rye. Gluten is the sticky part of the flour. The illustration on the following page may help you to understand just why the child with celiac disease cannot absorb gluten.

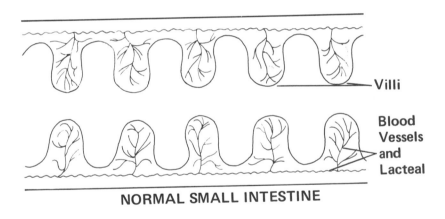

Villi

Blood Vessels and Lacteal

NORMAL SMALL INTESTINE

The normal small intestine contains small fingerlike structures on the inner lining called villi, which increase the amount of surface that can absorb the amino acids (completely digested proteins) and sugars into the blood vessel that runs down the center of the villus (singular). The fats are absorbed into the lacteal, which is in the center of the villus. These villi cause the food to be absorbed into the body at a rapid rate because of the large surface area they provide. The sugars, amino acids, and fats are then used to nourish the entire body and produce energy.

When a child has a celiac condition there is a lack of certain enzymes and the gluten in the wheat causes the cells in the villi to flatten. The exact reason for this flattening is unknown, however, doctors feel it is due most likely to destruction and

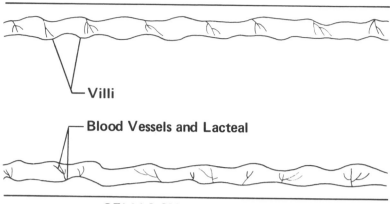

CELIAC SMALL INTESTINE

sloughing off of the villi caused by gluten irritation. Inflammation of the tissue could also account for some of the flattening. When these villi are missing, food that is passing through the intestine at the normal rate is not absorbed as fast as it should be because there is not enough surface area to do the job. This might be compared to wringing out a water-soaked sponge (normal intestine) and wringing out a water-soaked cloth (celiac intestine). Which contained the most water? The sponge did, because it has more absorbtive surface area.

When the waste products in the bowel are eliminated, the normal intestine has removed most of the nourishment but the celiac intestine has left much of the nourishment in the waste material. This may seem a hopeless situation to you, but you will find that if you faithfully eliminate the trouble-causing gluten from your child's diet, all of his symptoms will soon disappear and the child can live an otherwise perfectly normal existence.

In the past it was thought that the condition would be completely outgrown by the time a child reached adolescence, but recent research, according to Michael Gracy, M.D., M.R.A.C.P., head of the Gastro-Intestinal Research Unit of the Princess Margaret Children's Medical Research Foundation in Perth, Australia, has shown, "that this can lead to ill health and an increased incidence of gastro-intestinal cancer in later life. This has made mandatory the life-long exclusions of gluten from the diet of patients in which the disgnosis has been correctly established."

Since theirs is such a permanent life-style for the celiac patient it is important, for your child's and your own benefit, to have diagnostic tests run as soon as possible so that the proper treatment can be carried out.

The most important test is the duodenal biopsy which involves removal and microscopic examination of a tiny bit of the small intestine. Your doctor can give you a thorough explanation of the procedure, which gives a positive diagnosis of any type of malabsorption syndrome.

After the specific kind of allergy or malabsorption problem has been identified, your next task is becoming aware of the areas of your child's life that must be modified to maintain control of his condition.

3

It's a Part of Life

Every child, allergic or not, goes through basically the same joys and sorrows, trials and tribulations in life. The allergic child must often have his life-style altered to work around his allergies. If this can be done with a minimum of fuss it will give him a much more smoothly running childhood and prevent him from feeling, as much as possible, that he is different from other children who do not suffer from allergies.

Be sure that your pediatrician is aware of your child's allergies. Preventive immunizations are a routine part of every child's existence, and should be done at your doctor's discretion; but, it is essential to be sure the culture medium used for the vaccine is not one to which your child is allergic. There are many brands of the same vaccine which use a different culture as a base. The following list will help you determine possible allergens in immunization material.

1. Rubeola (Measles)—measle vaccine is grown in a chick embryo culture, which means egg. Two other culture media, rabbit and dog kidney, may be used.

2. Rubella (German Measles)—the cultures are bird, rabbit, dog, human or other mammal tissues.

3. DPT (Diphtheria, Whooping Cough, Tetanus)—the culture medium is beef broth. Alum is added to the serum to delay the absorption of the serum by the body. A new semi-synthetic culture medium inactivated with formaldehyde is also being used.

4. Mumps—cultured on chick embryo (egg).

5. Poliomyelitis—cultured on rhesus monkey kidney tissue and human tissue.

6. Influenza—grown on egg culture.

7. Typhus—grown on egg culture.

8. Smallpox—this vaccination is seldom given routinely today, but is often required for overseas travel. Cultured on calf lymph tissue or chick embryo.

9. Tetanus—horse serum.

10. Rabies Vaccine—cultured on duck embryo.

11. Typhoid—a sterile suspension in isotonic saline (salt) solution or suitable dilutent of killed typhoid bacilli.

12. Yellow Fever—chick embryo (egg).
13. Cholera—cultured in isotonic saline solution.

Most children have mild reactions to immunizations that are not the same as allergic reactions. Normal reactions might be crankiness, slightly elevated temperature, discomfort at the injection site, mild rash, or generalized malaise. The nurse or doctor who gives the injection will tell you what kind of reaction, if any, to expect from each type of immunization. If she does not, ask.

If your child has an unusual reaction such as diarrhea, vomiting, asthmatic attack, hives, hay fever symptoms, temperature over 101 degrees F. or convulsions, notify your doctor immediately.

Contagious diseases are part of the early lives of most children. In the event that your child is exposed to any of the childhood diseases that he has not been immunized against, it is helpful to know how long it will be before you should expect him to exhibit symptoms of the disease and be contagious himself. The following chart should help.

CONTAGIOUS DISEASES

Disease	Method of Spread	Incubation
Chicken Pox	Airborne virus—exposed day before symptoms appear or during symptoms	14-16 days
Diphtheria	Nasal and oral secretions and respiratory droplets of human cases and carriers. Food contaminated by above.	2-5 days
German Measles (Rubella)	Probably respiratory droplets of early cases (often the day before breaking out)	10-22 days, average 18
Influenza	Airborne Virus and human cases	18-36 hours
Measles (Rubeola)	Nasal and oral secretions of human cases and infected food	11-14 days
Tetanus	Horse and cattle feces and contaminated soil (contaminated puncture wound)	5 days to 5 weeks—average 10 days

Typhoid Fever	Infected urine and feces. Contaminated food and water.	5-14 days
Whooping Cough (Pertussis)	Infected bronchial secretions of human cases	12-20 days

Since all children become sick at one time or another and mothers of allergic children have even more reason than most to panic at the thought, some words of comfort may be in order to help calm the fears of a few mothers.

Caring for a sick child who is also allergic is not really any more difficult than caring for a nonallergic child. The most important point to remember is to keep the normal symptoms of the disease as mild as possible and to anticipate (but not imagine) possible complications. Here the old adage about an ounce of prevention being worth a pound of cure is certainly true. A cold could become pneumonia very easily in an asthmatic child if it is not cared for properly in the beginning. A slice of dry toast for a child with diarrhea caused by the flu could cause severe problems for an already inflammed gastrointestinal tract in a child who is allergic to milk and gluten.

You can see that it is vitally important to continue to follow your child's diet with modifications according to your doctor's advice. Don't give your child ginger ale (if he is allergic to citrus) just because the pediatrician's nurse said it was their standard treatment. She may know little or nothing of allergy problems and your child could have a reaction to the citric acid and corn syrup in the ginger ale and end up with diarrhea which isn't even a symptom of the measles. Now you have two problems to cope with! One caused by the virus and one caused by Mother.

Since many allergic children go to an allergist for their allergy problems and a pediatrician or general family doctor for illness and physical examinations, it is very important for the child's mother to keep on her toes. Be sure that your pediatrician is aware of all medications that your child takes routinely for his allergy. The size of the dosage and frequency is important too. An illustration of the importance of this is in the case of chicken pox. Doctors often prescribe medication to stop the itching. The medication usually given happens to be an antihistamine. If your child is already taking an antihistamine for his allergic runny nose, he could get an overdose.

Many mothers know home remedies for specific illnesses which must not be used with an allergic child. For example, giving orange juice for a cold, ginger ale for vomiting, popsicles for a sore throat. All of these contain citrus and possibly corn syrup. The consequences could be diarrhea, vomiting, rash or an asthma attack just because you allowed your child to go off his diet during an illness.

It is amazing, and rather frightening, to realize how much the life of an allergic child is dependent on medication, and how often we as parents know so little about the contents of the medications.

I have found with my own family that it is really most helpful to have one pharmacist who fills most of our prescriptions. When this is the case he becomes familiar with the medications that your child is taking and will know if a new prescription contains an ingredient which could cause difficulty when taken along with an already prescribed continuous medication. He can also quite often tell you if a medication contains one of your child's allergens. It is very important to have the pharmacist label all of your prescription bottles with the drug name. Not just the child's medications, but every prescription bottle that enters your home, as children do sometimes inadvertently obtain medication not intended for them.

Since we are discussing medication this is an excellent opportunity to stress drug safety. Keep all medications in a locked cabinet. Toddlers have a tendency to eat whatever they find in a bottle. Allergic children have an even greater tendency to do this, since they are given medication much more often. We learned this the hard way.

Our two-year-old was complaining of a tummy ache (not unusual for him since the majority of his problems were gastrointestinal). I gave him his prescribed medication but he still hurt, still insisted on aspirin "to make me feel better." I refused him and told him that his own medicine would help soon.

About ten minutes later I realized that the house was much too quiet. Upon investigating I found our little boy eating the last of a new bottle of baby aspirin. He had climbed to the top shelf of the linen closet, pulled down the box of aspirin, opened it, removed the safety cap, removed the cotton and eaten the entire contents. Fortunately, I had always kept a poison control kit on hand and after calling the doctor was able to give syrup of ipecac (which causes vomiting) immediately and then rush to the hospital. His initial blood tests indicated a high salicylate level and caused considerable concern, but quick treatment had eliminated much of the ingested aspirin and his blood test results soon began to return to normal. He was able to come home that night, but you can bet that our medicines were kept more than just "out of reach" after that!

Empty medicine containers may look like fascinating and harmless toys, but they can be as deadly as time bombs. This is especially true of a child with a chronic illness who is used to taking medication. Parents aren't the only ones guilty of giving children such dangerous "toys."

A three-year-old girl was given, by her doctor, a cute replica of scales that had at one time contained diet pills. She enjoyed this toy tremendously at his office but while playing soon realized that those little holes in the top of the scales were meant to hold pills. So! When she arrived home she filled them with aspirin and then proceeded to eat them. Her precocity and inventiveness were nearly fatal. Never underestimate the curiosity, ability, imagination and determination of a child!

Finding suitable toys for the allergic child can often cause concern, especially if he has contact allergies or has a habit of putting everything in his mouth.

Some of the toys that might cause difficulty are:

1. Dry clay—dust

2. Dry tempera paint—dust

3. Chalk—dust
4. Tents made from blankets—lint, dust
5. Twine macramé—lint from jute plant
6. Glue—fish, milk, or corn allergy
7. Sticker books—glue often contains corn
8. Stamp collecting—ditto
9. Wallpaper paste used with papier mache—wheat
10. Play dough—wheat or corn
11. Finger paints—corn
12. Crayons—dyes
13. Construction paper—dyes
14. Water colors—dyes
15. Marking pencils—dyes
16. India ink—dyes

But there is no need to assume that the joys of these toys must be totally forbidden to your child. There are several ways to adapt the toys to suit your circumstances.

Try making a washable percale tent to put over a card table. Be sure the trim is washable also.

Play dough can be made without wheat or dye using the following recipe:

PLAY DOUGH

1 ¼ cup rice flour
1   cup water
 ½ cup salt
1   tablespoon cooking oil
2   teaspoons cream of tartar (important)
Few drops of food coloring (optional)
Few drops of oil of wintergreen, cloves, cinnamon or vanilla for aroma

1. Mix dry ingredients in a heavy pan.
2. Add oil, water and food coloring to above.
3. Cook 3 minutes, stirring constantly, or until the mixture pulls away from the sides of the pan.
4. Add scent.
5. Knead lightly when cool enough, almost immediately.
6. Store in airtight container.

If you have an older child who is just starting to outgrow play dough (and you don't mind cleaning up a mess) here is one of my play dough experiment failures, that my girls, the neighborhood children, and my daughter's third-grade class really enjoyed and talked about for weeks. They named it:

THE BLOB

½ cup tapioca starch
1   cup water
½ cup salt
1   tablespoon cooking oil
2   teaspoons cream of tartar
Few drops of oil of wintergreen, cloves, cinnamon or vanilla for aroma
1. Mix dry ingredients in a heavy pan.
2. Add oil, water and scent to above.
3. Cook, stirring constantly until mixture pulls away from sides of pan (almost immediately).

This sticks to your hands but the children all thought it was worth it. When you pull it, it snaps back. It can be tipped upside down in your hand and pulled and it snaps back to the top hand. It feels like hard Jell-O and is very wiggly. I would suggest making this a "use-out-of-doors" plaything, with a pan of soapy water nearby to wash hands. It can be stored in a covered plastic container for about a month.

Finger-painting can be done on shelf paper with home-made finger-paints that do not contain cornstarch.

FINGER-PAINT

½ cup tapioca starch
½ cup cold water
1 ½ cups boiling water
½ cup Ivory flakes
1   tablespoon glycerin
Food coloring to desired color
1. Dissolve tapioca starch in the cold water.
2. Add the boiling water and cook the mixture until it is clear, stirring constantly.
3. Add the soap flakes and stir well.
4. Remove from stove immediately and cool.
5. Stir in glycerin and food coloring.

Making your own soap bubbles can give a child hours of joy.

BUBBLE STUFF

2 ⅔ cup Ivory flakes (not detergent)
1   teaspoon sugar
4   teaspoons glycerine (drugstore)
Pour the above ingredients into a quart jar with a lid and shake well. Fill the jar all but half an inch with lukewarm water. Screw the lid on tightly and shake very

hard. This mixture can be stored in the refrigerator but makes the best bubbles at room temperature or warmer. If you don't have a plastic bubble blower, a wooden spool can be used but blow lightly on spool. If you encounter any difficulty with the bubbles breaking before they are formed, add a bit more glycerin.

Most glues contain fish or corn; however, paste can usually be used without difficulty.

Paint-with-water books are always a good substitute for messy two-year-olds who cannot be trusted with crayons.

These are all good projects for those days that allergic children have more often than others; when they can't go out to play and need some new amusement to keep them happily occupied.

Feeding and amusing an allergic child in his own home is one thing, but what happens when he's not at home? Are you planning a trip or an outing? Go ahead! Here is a check list that may help you.

1. Check with your doctor if your child is on medication or allergy shots. He will arrange for you to have an adequate supply of serum and instructions for its administration.

2. Don't be afraid to take your child out to eat at a restaurant after his diet is regulated. It is a real treat for him, and for you. Just order plain broiled meats and baked or french fried potatoes. Stay away from hot dogs and hamburgers; they often contain ingredients that are not allowed on his diet. Ask to have his food left unbuttered, unfloured and without lemon on his fish. Just say that he has a special diet—you don't have to explain the entire problem. Restaurants are usually very cooperative. Be sure to remove anything your child cannot have from his plate. We have gone on two-week trips and eaten at restaurants the entire time with no difficulty.

3. Rice wafers, salted or unsalted (salted taste better) make a good cracker or bread substitute and don't need special storage. We take these to restaurants with us so our son doesn't feel left out when the rest of the family has crackers at the beginning of the meal.

4. Keep a few convenience packs of any allowable juice on hand to take with you when you eat out. Also buy small individual jars of applesauce or other fruit for desserts.

5. If you have room in the car, take a cooler chest for formula, fruit, celery sticks, etc. This helps extinguish that between-meal hunger. It also relieves your mind as to whether your allergic child is getting enough to eat. Relax and enjoy your trip, and he will too!

A few days in the hospital can present a real problem for the food-allergic child. I know! Our son was hospitalized three times in his first two years. Much apprehension on your part can be avoided if you are aware of the following:

1. Doctors, especially surgeons who don't see your child normally, are used to writing orders for regular diets without restricting particular foods. The hospital dietitians only give the diet that the doctor orders. It is important that your doctor

knows *before* the child is hospitalized that he requires an allergy diet, since orders often reach the hospital before the patient.

2. Bring with you from home two copies of your list of allowed and disallowed foods. One list goes on the chart at the nurses' station and the other goes to the dietitian.

3. When you arrive on the floor where your child is to be cared for, request an appointment with the dietitian.

4. The dietitian will tell you what she can provide for your child from the hospital supplies. Usually they *will not* cook special treats for an allergic child. The best thing to do is to ask if you may bring a specific treat to be kept in his bedside stand or the floor refrigerator. Don't forget to label any snacks that you bring in, with your child's name and room and bed number in large print! Remember not to give treats without knowing if the diet has been further restricted. For example, the child may be on a clear liquid diet after surgery. Don't just assume that you know best. Ask and be sure.

5. Try to be at the hospital as much as allowed, especially if your child is a toddler. If you can't be there when food would most likely be passed out, leave notes. A strip of adhesive tape at the head of the bed that reads: "ALLERGY DIET—SEE CHART" would be helpful to those working with your child. Also, if he is allowed out of bed, place the same warning on his robe or pajamas with a strip of tape.

6. The aide who is working with your child should be told that he has restrictions as to snacks and milk. Nurse's aides sometimes tend to treat all children alike when passing out snacks. Often milk is accidentally sent with cereal on allergy trays and aides just assume that it is all right unless they are told otherwise ahead of time.

As you can see, the life of an allergic child need not be that of an invalid who must at all costs be kept confined to his own little world, eliminating all the joys of childhood. I know that you want your child's life to be as normal as possible. This can be accomplished by just enjoying your child and allowing him to experience all of the life that your family enjoys—he need not be an outcast.

Nutrition is something every good mother needs to know about, but to juggle the diet of an allergic child demands an even greater understanding of how food nourishes our bodies.

4

What Eating is All About

Nothing worries a parent more than a child who isn't getting enough to eat, even if it is just a toddler who is temporarily going through a "phase." The parent of a child with food allergies tends to worry even more. Even if his child does eat, there is the ever-present obligation to deny him some of the most nutritious foods because of his allergic reactions to them. Therefore, working with an allergy diet requires a basic understanding of nutrition.

There are three types of nutrients that provide adequate nutrition and the calories that are needed by your child for growth, repair, and maintenance of his body. These are proteins, carbohydrates, and fats. The allergic child may require a higher than usual intake of all nutrients because of susceptibility to infection, interference with normal intestinal absorption of the nutrients, and allergic reactions. For example, the comparison of an allergic and nonallergic child's usual protein consumption shows the allergic child's to be much greater.

Protein is a basic building block of the human body and the need for it is greatest in infancy since a child can be expected to double or triple his weight during the first year of life. The protein needs per pound of body weight decrease gradually as the child grows, until, as an adult, protein is needed primarily to repair and rebuild cells. The body uses protein not only to build muscles, skin, hair, nerve tissue, blood components, and body tissues in general, but also to repair any of these when damaged due to injury, sickness, or infection.

The adequacy of protein intake in the diet is most often measured by the growth in height of the child. However, if the intake of carbohydrate or total calories is too low, protein will be used, although inefficiently, for energy, and growth may be slowed.

Protein is provided mainly by milk (or prepared formulas that are similar in nutritive content to milk), meat, fish, eggs, cheese, and dried beans and peas. Grain products and starch vegetables such as corn and potatoes contribute small amounts of protein. The amounts to be found in the "Basic Four" food groups can be seen in the charts on page 40.

Carbohydrates are the main energy supply for the body. They may be complex compounds such as are found in dried beans, potatoes and bread, or they can be the simple sugars found in milk and fruit.

The body stores extra carbohydrate so that it can be mobilized in case of illness or allergic reactions. However it is still important for the child to be given carbohydrate during illness or reactions because his energy needs at these crucial times are increased. The carbohydrates may be given along with the fluids that he is able to tolerate.

The minimum amount of carbohydrate needed per day by an adult is 100 grams, which would be found in two cups of milk, four slices of bread (or cereal substitutes), and two servings of fruit or fruit juice. A child will need even more.

Fats are a much more concentrated source of energy than carbohydrates. They are digested more slowly than protein or carbohydrate and provide a satisfied, full feeling to the diet. If the physician prescribes a diet low in fat, the energy normally supplied by fat will need to be supplied by increasing the amount of carbohydrate primarily, and also slightly increasing the amount of protein.

Besides being a source of energy, fats carry vitamins A, D, and E, and the fatlike substances used in the body to make hormones and digestive juices. Ingested fats help maintain a normal secretion of skin and hair oils. If the fat is not needed for energy, it is changed into fatty tissue which supports and protects vital organs such as the kidneys and liver. The adequacy of the fat tissue on the body can be determined by looking at the individual or consulting height-weight tables.

If the protein intake is high, the fat intake will usually be high, since meat is the primary source for protein in most diets and meat contains both protein and fat. Signs of inadequate fat intake can be skin changes similar to skin allergy reactions, and for this reason it is wise to check the allergic child's diet for fat content.

You will find that the diet contained in this book is adequate in protein, low in fat and consequently higher in carbohydrate in order to provide adequate calories as well as all essential nutrients to provide a well-balanced diet.

Since an allergy diet is necessarily restricted in the foods that are allowed, it is very important that you work out your child's diet to include as many of the basic four foods as possible. The chart which follows contains the foods required for a normal diet and is not intended for you to follow for your allergic child, for obvious reasons. The second chart is an adaptation of the first, and includes foods to be used for the allergic individual.

You will notice that your child's list of allowed foods eliminates many of the foods on the "Normal Daily Basic Four." Don't worry about this, just do the best you can and add new foods as often as the doctor permits. Give your child as much of the protein foods as he can tolerate and give him the vitamin supplement that your doctor has recommended. With this and the extra foods he eats during the day, he should be getting an adequate diet. (An important observation at this point: When a toddler is given meat cookies before ever tasting sweet cookies he enjoys them just as much. Once he discovers that cookies are supposed to be sweet, he may refuse to eat the high-protein, low-carbohydrate, meat cookies. Try the meat cookies first as a treat.)

"NORMAL DAILY BASIC FOUR"

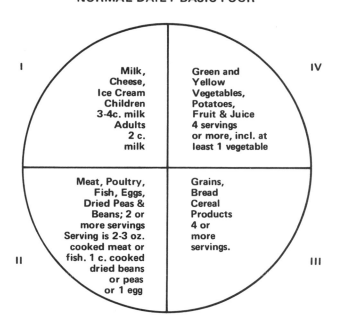

I

Milk,
Cheese,
Ice Cream
Children
3-4c. milk
Adults
2 c.
milk

Green and
Yellow
Vegetables,
Potatoes,
Fruit & Juice
4 servings
or more, incl. at
least 1 vegetable

IV

Meat, Poultry,
Fish, Eggs,
Dried Peas &
Beans; 2 or
more servings
Serving is 2-3 oz.
cooked meat or
fish. 1 c. cooked
dried beans
or peas
or 1 egg

Grains,
Bread
Cereal
Products
4 or
more
servings.

II   III

"SAMPLE ALLERGIC DAILY BASIC FOUR"

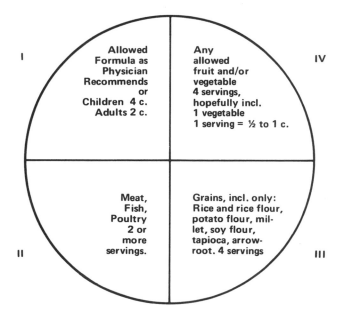

I

Allowed
Formula as
Physician
Recommends
or
Children 4 c.
Adults 2 c.

Any
allowed
fruit and/or
vegetable
4 servings,
hopefully incl.
1 vegetable
1 serving = ½ to 1 c.

IV

Meat,
Fish,
Poultry
2 or
more
servings.

Grains, incl. only:
Rice and rice flour,
potato flour, mil-
let, soy flour,
tapioca, arrow-
root. 4 servings

II   III

When you are first starting with your allergic child's diet, it is difficult to judge whether he is getting a sufficient quantity of all nutrients. Your best bet is to keep working slowly toward the goals on the Basic Four chart. An explanation of vitamins and minerals has been omitted from the nutrition section, not because they are unimportant, but because most doctors put a food-allergic child on a vitamin supplement to suit the child's individual needs. These supplements, plus formula, plus the foods that your child can tolerate, will give him an adequate vitamin and mineral intake.

So you can see more clearly what can be done with an allergy diet I will show you my son David's starting diet and his diet at age four. With his diet is a comparable diet for a three-year-old with no dietary restrictions.

DAVID'S STARTING DIET (Age eight months)
Soy base diluted—2 ounces formula to 6 ounces water
Raw scraped apple
Rice
Meat cookies
Knox gelatin
Apple juice
Pears
Beef, lamb, veal
Rice wafers

This limited list includes all of the food that David could tolerate at the beginning of his allergy diet. He ate these foods only for about two months until his gastrointestinal symptoms disappeared, and then foods were added one at a time, until he now has quite a lengthy list. (The following list is broken down into the Basic Four.

GROUP 1

Soy base
Soy base

GROUP 2

Beef
Lamb
Veal
Knox gelatin
Pork—fresh
Chicken—limited

GROUP 3

Rice
Millet
Rice wafers and cakes
Sesame seeds

GROUP 4

Apple
Pears
Apple juice
Bananas

GROUP 3 (cont.)   GROUP 4 (cont.)

Rice flour   Black Cherries
Soybean flour   Potatoes
Potato flour   Spinach
Tapioca starch flour   Lettuce
Grainless mix   Celery
                                             Green pepper
                                             Green beans
                                             Beets

Plus list in appendix of available brands of allowed food products

COMPARISON OF DIETS

Diet	Calories	Protein (grams)	Carbohydrate (grams)	Fat (grams)
David's	1948	74	310	74
Usual 2-3-Year-old's	1303	50	125	57
Recommended dietary allowances 2-3-year-old	1250	25		

COMPARABLE REGULAR DIET AT AGE 3 (SAMPLE)

BREAKFAST

	Calories	Protein	Carbohydrate	Fat
Orange juice ½ c.	55	1	14	trace
Corn flakes 1 c.	110	2	24	trace
Milk 1 c.	165	9	12	10

LUNCH

	Calories	Protein	Carbohydrate	Fat
Broiled chicken 1 oz.	38.3	616	—	1
Bread, white enriched 1 slice	60	2	11	1
Mayonnaise 1 teasp.	36.6	trace	trace	4
Carrot sticks, 2	1	trace	.2	trace
Celery sticks, 2	.5	trace	trace	trace
Milk, 1 c.	165	9	12	10
Chocolate chip cookies, 2	329	17	27	17

DINNER

Roast beef 2.3 oz., lean	115	19	–	4
Mashed potatoes, ½ c.	72.5	2	15	.5
Green beans, ½ c.	12.5	1	3	trace
Applesauce, ½ c.	92.5	–	25	–
Milk, 1 c.	165	9	12	10
Daily totals	1427.9	77.6	156.2	57.5

DAVID'S DIET AT AGE 3 (SAMPLE)

	Calories	Protein	Carbohydrate	Fat
BREAKFAST				
Apple juice, 1 cup.	125	trace	34	–
Rice Chex, 1 c.	95.2	1.3	20.8	0.08
Soy base 1:2 dilution				
½ c.	77.7	2.2	15.4	4.3
MIDMORNING SNACK				
Roasted soybean ½ c.				
approximately	345.8	34.6	29.8	98
LUNCH				
*Chicken-vegetable with				
rice soup—1 c.	152.8	16.4	18.1	1.3
*2" Rice flour pancakes, 2	16.1	.3	2.7	.6
Honey, 1 teasp.	60	trace	17	–
*Dutch apple ice, 1 c.	402.1	5.7	71.9	11.3
AFTERNOON SNACK				
*Applesauce cookies, 2	130	1.4	22.2	2.1
Soy base 1:2 Dil. 1 c.	155.3	4.3	15.4	8.5
DINNER				
*Leg of lamb, 3 oz.	265	20	–	20
Green beans, ½ c.	12.5	1	3	trace
*Mashed potatoes, ½ c.	90	3	21	trace
Apple juice, 1 c.	125	trace	34	–
Applesauce, ½ c.	92.5	–	25	–
Daily totals	2144.9	90.2	330.3	146.18

*Recipe in this book

By comparing the diets that have gone before, you will be better able to see just where the differences, as well as the similarities, lie. You can see that with imagination and common sense, your allergic child can have a perfectly adequate, balanced, appetizing diet.

To assist you in your diet planning, the following pages contain a wonderfully complete list of foods with the nutrient amounts carefully broken down. These nutrient tables were provided by the United States Department of Agriculture.

Explanation of the Table

The values shown in the table that follows are in terms of common units of measure, as one cup, one ounce, or a piece of specified size. The quantities of foods thus shown can be converted readily to particular serving portions. The one-cup amount, for example, can be reduced or multiplied in estimating servings of various sizes.

The cup measure used refers to the standard 8-ounce measuring cup of 8 fluid ounces or one-half liquid pint. The ounce shown is by weight, that is, one-sixteenth of a pound avoirdupois, unless the fluid ounce is indicated.

Most of the foods listed in the table are in ready-to-serve form, but a few items frequently used as ingredients in prepared dishes have been included.

Values for many of the food mixtures have been calculated from typical recipes. The cooked vegetables have no added fat.

A column showing water content is in the table, as the percentage of moisture is frequently useful in identifying and comparing food items.

Parts of some foods, as seeds, skins, bone, are either inedible or may be eaten but usually are discarded. The nutrient values in the table apply to the parts customarily eaten. Values for potato, for example, apply to potato without the skin. If the skin also is eaten, the amounts of some nutrients will be a little larger than shown in the table.

Nutrients in Common Foods in Terms of Household Measures

Item number	Food	Water	Food energy	Protein	Fat	Total carbohydrate	Calcium	Iron	Vitamin A value	Thiamine	Riboflavin	Niacin	Ascorbic acid
		Per cent	Calories	Grams	Grams	Grams	Milligrams	Milligrams	International Units	Milligrams	Milligrams	Milligrams	Milligrams
	MILK AND MILK PRODUCTS												
	Milk; 1 cup:												
1	Fluid, whole	87	165	9	10	12	285	0.1	390	0.08	0.42	0.2	2
2	Fluid, nonfat (skim)	90	90	9	Trace	13	298	.1	10	.10	.44	.2	2
3	Buttermilk, cultured (from skim milk)	90	90	9	Trace	13	298	.1	10	.10	.44	.2	2
4	Evaporated (undiluted)	74	345	18	20	24	635	.3	820	.10	.84	.5	3
5	Condensed, sweetened (undiluted)	26	985	25	25	170	829	.3	1,020	.24	1.21	.5	3
6	Dry, whole	2	515	27	28	39	968	.5	1,160	.30	1.50	.7	6
7	Dry, nonfat	3	290	29	1	42	1,040	.5	20	.28	1.44	.7	6
8	Half and half (milk and cream)	80	330	8	29	11	259	.1	1,190	.07	.39	.1	2
	Cream; 1 tablespoon:												
9	Light, table or coffee	72	30	Trace	3	1	15	Trace	120	Trace	.02	Trace	Trace
10	Heavy or whipping	59	50	Trace	5	Trace	12	Trace	220	Trace	.02	Trace	Trace
	Milk beverages; 1 cup:												
11	Cocoa (all milk)	79	235	9	11	26	286	.9	390	.09	.45	.4	2
12	Chocolate flavored drink	83	190	8	6	27	270	.4	210	.09	.41	.2	2
13	Malted milk	78	280	12	12	32	364	.8	680	.18	.56	.....	3
14	Yogurt (from partially skimmed milk); 1 cup	89	120	8	4	13	295	.1	170	.09	.43	.2	2
	Cheese; 1 ounce:												
15	Cheddar, or American	36	115	7	9	1	221	.3	380	.01	.15	Trace	0
16	Cheddar, processed	39	105	7	9	Trace	214	.2	350	Trace	.12	Trace	0
17	Cheese foods, Cheddar	43	95	6	7	2	163	.2	300	.01	.17	Trace	0
	Cottage:												
18	From skim milk	79	25	5	Trace	1	26	.1	Trace	.01	.08	Trace	0
19	Creamed	78	30	4	1	1	25	.1	50	.01	.08	Trace	0
20	Cream cheese	51	105	2	11	Trace	18	.2	440	Trace	.07	Trace	0
21	Roquefort, or blue	40	105	6	9	1	122	.3	350	.01	.17	.1	0
22	Swiss	39	105	7	8		271		320	.01	.06	Trace	0
	Desserts (largely milk):												
23	Cornstarch pudding, plain; 1 cup	76	275	9	10	39	290	.1	390	.07	.40	.1	2
24	Custard, baked; 1 cup, 8 fluid ounces	77	285	13	14	28	278	1.0	870	.10	.47	.2	1

No.	Food												
	Ice cream, plain, factory packed:												
25	1 slice or individual brick, ½ quart	62	165	3	10	17	100	.1	420	.03	.15	.1	1
26	1 container, 3½ fluid ounces	62	130	2	8	13	76	.1	320	.03	.12	.1	1
27	1 container, 8 fluid ounces	62	295	6	18	29	175	.1	740	.06	.27	.1	1
28	Ice milk; 1 cup, 8 fluid ounces	67	285	9	10	42	292	.2	420	.09	.41	.2	2

EGGS

No.	Food												
	Egg, raw, large:												
29	1 whole	74	80	6	6	Trace	27	1.1	590	.05	.15	Trace	0
30	1 white	88	15	4	Trace	Trace	3	Trace	0	Trace	.09	Trace	0
31	1 yolk	51	60	3	5	Trace	24	.9	580	.04	.07	Trace	0
	Egg, cooked; 1 large:												
32	Boiled	74	80	6	6	Trace	27	1.1	590	.05	.14	Trace	0
33	Scrambled (with milk and fat)	72	110	7	8	1	51	1.1	690	.05	.18	Trace	0

MEAT, POULTRY, FISH, SHELLFISH

No.	Food												
34	Bacon, broiled or fried, medium done; 2 slices	13	95	4	9	Trace	4	.5	0	.08	.05	.8	0
	Beef, cooked, without bone:												
	Braised, simmered, or pot-roasted; 3-ounce portion:												
35	Entire portion, lean and fat	43	340	20	28	0	9	2.6	50	.04	.15	3.1	0
36	Lean only, approx. 2 ounces	62	115	18	4	0	8	2.2	Trace	.03	.13	2.7	0
	Hamburger patties, made with—												
37	Regular ground beef; 3-ounce patty	54	245	21	17	0	9	2.7	30	.07	.02	4.6	0
38	Lean ground round; 3-ounce patty	60	185	23	10	0	10	3.0	20	.08	.20	5.1	0
	Roast; 3-ounce slice from—												
	Cut having relatively large amount of fat:												
39	Entire portion, lean and fat	35	420	15	39	0	7	2.0	80	.04	.12	2.8	0
40	Lean only, approx. 1.6 ounces	57	110	13	6	0	6	1.7	Trace	.03	.10	2.4	0
	Cut having relatively small amount of fat:												
41	Entire portion, lean and fat	52	255	22	18	0	9	2.8	30	.06	.16	3.9	0
42	Lean only, approx. 2.3 ounces	63	115	19	4	0	8	2.4	Trace	.05	.14	3.4	0

Nutrients in Common Foods in Terms of Household Measures—Continued

Item number	Food	Water	Food energy	Protein	Fat	Total carbohydrate	Calcium	Iron	Vitamin A value	Thiamine	Riboflavin	Niacin	Ascorbic acid
		Per cent	Calories	Grams	Grams	Grams	Milligrams	Milligrams	International Units	Milligrams	Milligrams	Milligrams	Milligrams
	MEAT, POULTRY, FISH, SHELL-FISH—Con.												
	Beef, cooked, without bone—Con.												
	Steak, broiled; 3-ounce portion:												
43	Entire portion, lean and fat...	39	375	19	32	0	9	2.6	60	0.06	0.16	4.0	0
44	Lean only, approx. 1.8 ounces..	59	105	17	4	0	7	2.0	Trace	.05	.13	3.3	0
	Beef, canned:												
45	Corned; 3 ounces...	59	180	22	10	0	17	3.7	20	.01	.20	2.9	0
46	Corned beef hash; 3 ounces...	70	120	12	5	6	22	1.1	10	.02	.11	2.4	0
47	Beef, dried; 2 ounces...	48	115	19	4	0	11	2.9	......	.04	.18	2.2	0
48	Beef and vegetable stew; 1 cup...	79	250	13	19	17	31	2.6	2,520	.12	.15	3.4	15
	Chicken, without bone:												
49	Broiled; 3 ounces...	71	115	20	3	0	8	1.4	80	.06	.15	10.5	0
50	Canned; 3 ounces...	62	170	25	7	0	12	1.5	160	.03	.14	5.4	0
	Chile con carne, canned:												
51	Without beans; 1 cup...	67	510	26	38	15	97	3.6	380	.05	.31	5.6	......
52	Heart, beef, trimmed of fat, braised; 3 ounces...	61	160	26	5	1	14	5.9	30	.23	1.05	6.8	3
	Lamb, cooked:												
	Chops; 1 thick chop, with bone, 4.8 ounces:												
53	Lean and fat, approx. 3.6 ounces.	44	450	24	39	0	10	2.9	......	.13	.24	5.4	0
54	Lean only, 2.4 ounces...	62	130	19	5	0	8	2.3	......	.10	.19	4.2	0
	Roast, without bone:												
	Leg; 3-ounce slice:												
55	Entire slice, lean and fat...	51	265	20	20	0	9	2.6	......	.12	.22	4.5	0
56	Lean only, approx. 2.3 ounces...	62	120	19	5	0	9	2.4	......	.11	.20	4.1	0
	Shoulder; 3-ounce portion, without bone:												
57	Entire portion, lean and fat..	48	300	18	25	0	9	2.3	......	.11	.19	4.0	0
58	Lean only, approx. 2.2 ounces...	61	125	16	6	0	7	2.1	......	.09	.17	3.5	0

No.	Food												
59	Liver, beef, fried; 2 ounces	57	120	13	4	6	5	4.4	30,330	.15	2.25	8.4	18
60	Ham, smoked; 3-ounce portion, without bone	39	340	20	28	Trace	9	2.5	0	.46	.18	3.5	0
	Luncheon meat:												
61	Boiled ham; 2 ounces	48	170	13	13	0	5	1.5	0	.57	.15	2.9	0
62	Canned, spiced; 2 ounces	55	165	8	14	1	5	1.2	0	.18	.12	1.6	0
	Pork, fresh, cooked:												
	Chops; 1 chop, with bone, 3.5 ounces:												
63	Lean and fat, approx. 2.4 ounces	39	295	15	25	0	7	2.1	.....	.60	.17	3.6	0
64	Lean only, approx. 1.6 ounces	53	120	14	7	0	6	1.8	.....	.51	.15	3.1	0
	Roast; 3-ounce slice, without bone:												
65	Entire slice, lean and fat	43	340	19	29	0	9	2.5	.....	.71	.21	4.3	0
66	Lean only, approx. 2.2 ounces	55	160	19	9	0	8	2.4	.....	.68	.20	4.1	0
	Simmered; 3-ounce portion, without bone:												
67	Entire portion, lean and fat	42	355	19	30	0	9	2.4	.....	.43	.20	3.9	0
68	Lean only, approx. 2 ounces	60	120	16	5	0	7	2.0	.....	.37	.17	3.3	0
	Sausage:												
69	Bologna; 8 slices (4.1 by 0.1 inches each), 8 ounces	56	690	27	62	2	16	4.1	.....	.36	.49	6.0	0
70	Frankfurter; 1 cooked, 1.8 ounces	58	155	6	14	1	3	.8	.....	.08	.10	1.3	0
71	Pork, bulk, canned; 4 ounces	55	340	18	29	0	10	2.6	.....	.23	.27	3.4	0
72	Tongue, beef, boiled or simmered; 3 ounces	61	205	18	14	Trace	7	2.5	.....	.04	.26	3.1	0
73	Veal, cutlet, broiled; 3-ounce portion, without bone	60	185	23	9	0	9	2.7	.....	.06	.21	4.6	0
	Fish and shellfish:												
74	Bluefish, baked or broiled; 3 ounces	68	135	22	4	0	25	.6	40	.09	.08	1.6	0
	Clams:												
75	Raw, meat only; 3 ounces	80	70	11	1	3	82	6.0	90	.08	.15	1.4	0
76	Canned, solids and liquid; 3 ounces	87	45	7	1	2	74	5.4	70	.04	.08	.9	0
77	Crabmeat, canned or cooked; 3 ounces	77	90	14	2	1	38	.8	.....	.04	.05	2.1	0
78	Fishsticks, breaded, cooked, frozen; 10 sticks (3.8 by 1.0 by 0.5 inches each), 8 ounces	66	400	38	20	15	25	.9	.....	.09	.16	3.6	0
79	Haddock, fried; 3 ounces	67	135	16	5	6	15	.5	50	.03	.08	2.2	0

Nutrients in Common Foods in Terms of Household Measures—Continued

Item number	Food	Water (Per cent)	Food energy (Calories)	Protein (Grams)	Fat (Grams)	Total carbohydrate (Grams)	Calcium (Milligrams)	Iron (Milligrams)	Vitamin A value (International Units)	Thiamine (Milligrams)	Riboflavin (Milligrams)	Niacin (Milligrams)	Ascorbic acid (Milligrams)
	MEAT, POULTRY, FISH, SHELLFISH—Con.												
	Fish and shellfish—Continued												
	Mackerel:												
80	Broiled; 3 ounces	62	200	19	13	0	5	1.0	40	0.13	0.23	6.5	0
81	Canned, solids and liquid; 3 ounces	66	155	16	9	0	157	1.8	370	.05	.18	4.9	0
82	Ocean perch, fried (dipped in egg and bread crumbs); 3 ounces	59	195	16	11	6	14	1.3	50	.09	.10	1.7	0
	Oysters, raw, meat only; 1 cup (13–												
83	19 medium-size oysters, selects)	85	160	20	4	8	226	13.2	740	.30	.39	6.6	0
84	Oyster stew; 1 cup (6–8 oysters)	84	200	11	12	11	269	3.3	640	.12	.40	1.7	0
85	Salmon, canned (pink); 3 ounces	70	120	17	5	0	159	.7	60	.03	.16	6.8	0
	Sardines, canned in oil, drained												
86	solids; 3 ounces	57	180	22	9	1	367	2.5	190	.02	.18	4.6	0
87	Shad, baked; 3 ounces	64	170	20	10	0	20	.5	20	.11	.22	7.3	......
	Shrimp, canned, meat only; 3												
88	ounces	66	110	23	1	......	98	2.6	50	.01	.03	1.9	0
89	Swordfish; 3 ounces	65	150	24	5	0	23	1.1	1,750	.03	.04	9.3	0
	Tuna, canned in oil, drained solids;												
90	3 ounces	60	170	25	7	0	7	1.2	70	.04	.10	10.9	0
	MATURE BEANS AND PEAS: NUTS												
91	Almonds, shelled; 1 cup	5	850	26	77	28	332	6.7	0	.34	1.31	5.0	Trace
	Beans, dry seed:												
	Common varieties, as Great Northern, navy, and others, canned; 1 cup:												
92	Red	76	230	15	1	42	74	4.6	0	.13	.13	1.5	Trace
	White, with tomato or molasses:												
93	With pork	69	330	16	7	54	172	4.4	140	.13	.10	1.3	5
94	Without pork	69	315	16	1	60	183	5.2	140	.13	.10	1.3	5

No.	Food												
95	Lima, cooked; 1 cup	64	260	16	1	48	56	5.6	Trace	.26	.12	1.3	Trace
96	Brazil nuts, broken pieces; 1 cup	5	905	20	92	15	260	4.8	Trace	1.21	.....	.....	.....
97	Cashew nuts, roasted; 1 cup	5	770	25	65	35	51	5.1	.....	.49	.46	1.9	.....
	Coconut; 1 cup:												
98	Fresh, shredded	50	330	3	31	13	15	1.7	0	.06	.03	.5	4
99	Dried, shredded (sweetened)	3	345	2	24	33	13	1.6	0	.04	.02	.4	0
100	Cowpeas or black-eyed peas, dry, cooked; 1 cup	80	190	13	1	34	42	3.2	20	.41	.11	1.1	Trace
101	Peanuts, roasted, shelled; 1 cup	2	840	39	71	28	104	3.2	0	.47	.19	24.6	0
102	Peanut butter; 1 tablespoon	2	90	4	8	3	12	.4	0	.02	.02	2.8	0
103	Peas, split, dry, cooked; 1 cup	70	290	20	1	52	28	4.2	120	.36	.22	2.2	Trace
104	Pecans, halves; 1 cup	3	740	10	77	16	79	2.6	140	.93	.14	1.0	2
	Walnuts, shelled; 1 cup:												
105	Black or native, chopped	3	790	26	75	19	Trace	7.6	380	.28	.14	.9	.....
106	English or Persian, halves	4	650	15	64	16	99	3.1	30	.33	.13	.9	3

VEGETABLES

No.	Food												
	Asparagus:												
107	Cooked; 1 cup	92	35	4	Trace	6	33	1.8	1,820	.23	.30	2.1	40
	Canned; 6 medium-size spears:												
108	Green	92	20	2	Trace	3	18	1.8	770	.06	.08	.9	17
109	Bleached	92	20	2	Trace	4	15	1.0	70	.05	.07	.8	17
	Beans:												
110	Lima, immature, cooked; 1 cup	75	150	8	1	29	46	2.7	460	.22	.14	1.8	24
	Snap, green:												
	Cooked; 1 cup:												
111	In small amount of water, short time	92	25	2	Trace	6	45	.9	830	.09	.12	.6	18
112	In large amount of water, long time	92	25	2	Trace	6	45	.9	830	.06	.11	.5	12
	Canned:												
113	Solids and liquid; 1 cup	94	45	2	Trace	10	65	3.3	990	.08	.10	.7	9
114	Strained or chopped; 1 ounce	93	5	Trace	Trace	1	10	.3	120	.01	.02	.1	1
115	Beets, cooked, diced; 1 cup	88	70	2	Trace	16	35	1.2	30	.03	.07	.5	11
116	Broccoli, cooked, flower stalks; 1 cup	90	45	5	Trace	8	195	2.0	5,100	.10	.22	1.2	111
117	Brussels sprouts, cooked; 1 cup	85	60	6	1	12	44	1.7	520	.05	.16	.6	61
	Cabbage; 1 cup:												
118	Raw, finely shredded	92	25	1	Trace	5	46	.5	80	.06	.05	.3	50
119	Raw, coleslaw	84	100	2	7	9	47	.5	80	.06	.05	.3	50

Nutrients in Common Foods in Terms of Household Measures—Continued

Item number	Food	Water	Food energy	Protein	Fat	Total carbohydrate	Calcium	Iron	Vitamin A value	Thiamine	Riboflavin	Niacin	Ascorbic acid
		Per cent	Calories	Grams	Grams	Grams	Milligrams	Milligrams	International Units	Milligrams	Milligrams	Milligrams	Milligrams
	VEGETABLES—Con.												
	Cabbage; 1 cup—Con.												
	Cooked:												
120	In small amount of water, short time	92	40	2	Trace	9	78	0.8	150	0.08	0.08	0.5	53
121	In large amount of water, long time	92	40	2	Trace	9	78	.8	150	.05	.05	.3	32
	Cabbage, celery or Chinese; 1 cup:												
122	Raw, leaves and stem (1-inch pieces)	95	15	1	Trace	2	43	.9	260	.03	.04	.4	31
123	Cooked	95	25	2	1	5	82	1.7	490	.04	.06	.6	42
	Carrots:												
124	Raw; 1 carrot (5½ by 1 inch) or 25 thin strips	88	20	1	Trace	5	20	.4	6,000	.03	.03	.3	3
125	Raw, grated; 1 cup	88	45	1	Trace	10	43	.9	13,200	.06	.06	.7	7
126	Cooked, diced; 1 cup	92	45	1	1	9	38	.9	18,130	.07	.07	.7	6
127	Canned, strained or chopped; 1 ounce	92	5	Trace	0	2	7	.2	3,400	.01	.01	.1	1
128	Cauliflower, cooked, flower buds; 1 cup	92	30	3	Trace	6	26	1.3	110	.07	.10	.6	34
	Celery, raw:												
129	Large stalk, 8 inches long	94	5	1	Trace	1	20	.2	0	.02	.02	.2	3
130	Diced; 1 cup	94	20	1	Trace	4	50	.5	0	.05	.04	.4	7
131	Collards, cooked; 1 cup	87	75	7	1	14	473	3.0	14,500	.15	.46	3.2	84
	Corn, sweet:												
132	Cooked; 1 ear 5 inches long	76	65	2	1	16	4	.5	1,300	.09	.08	1.1	6
133	Canned, solids and liquid; 1 cup	80	170	5	1	41	10	1.3	1,520	.07	.13	2.4	14
134	Cowpeas, immature seeds, cooked; 1 cup	75	150	11	1	25	59	4.0	620	.46	.13	1.3	32
135	Cucumbers, raw, pared; 6 slices (⅛-inch thick, center section)	96	5	Trace	Trace	1	5	.2	0	.02	.02	.1	4
136	Dandelion greens, cooked; 1 cup	86	80	5	1	16	337	5.6	27,310	.23	.22	1.3	29
137	Endive, curly (including escarole); 2 ounces	93	10	1	Trace	2	45	1.0	1,700	.04	.07	.1	6
138	Kale, cooked; 1 cup	87	45	4	1	8	248	2.4	9,220	.08	.25	1.9	56

139	Lettuce, headed, raw: 2 large or 4 small leaves	95	5	1	Trace	1	11	.2	270	.02	.04	.1	4
140	1 compact head (4¾-inch diameter)	95	70	5	1	13	100	2.3	2,470	.20	.38	.9	35
141	Mushrooms, canned, solids and liquid; 1 cup	93	30	3	Trace	9	17	2.0	0	.04	.60	4.8	....
142	Mustard greens, cooked; 1 cup	92	30	3	Trace	6	308	4.1	10,050	.08	.25	1.0	63
143	Okra, cooked; 8 pods (3 inches long, ⅝-inch diameter)	90	30	2	Trace	6	70	.6	630	.05	.05	.7	17
	Onions: Mature:												
144	Raw; 1 onion (2½-inch diameter)	88	50	2	Trace	11	35	.6	60	.04	.04	.2	10
145	Cooked; 1 cup	90	80	2	Trace	18	67	1.0	110	.04	.06	.4	13
146	Young green; 6 small, without tops	88	25	Trace	Trace	5	68	.4	30	.02	.02	.1	12
147	Parsley, raw; 1 tablespoon chopped	84	1	Trace	Trace	Trace	7	.2	290	Trace	.01	.1	7
148	Parsnips, cooked; 1 cup	84	95	2	1	22	88	1.1	0	.09	.16	.3	19
	Peas, green; 1 cup:												
149	Cooked	82	110	8	1	19	35	3.0	1,150	.40	.22	3.7	24
150	Canned, solids and liquid	82	170	8	1	32	62	4.5	1,350	.28	.15	2.6	21
151	Canned, strained; 1 ounce	86	10	1	Trace	2	5	.3	160	.03	.02	.3	2
	Peppers, sweet:												
152	Green, raw; 1 medium	93	15	1	Trace	3	6	.4	260	.05	.05	.3	79
153	Red, raw; 1 medium	91	20	1	Trace	4	8	.4	2,670	.05	.05	.3	122
154	Pimientos, canned; 1 medium	92	10	Trace	Trace	2	3	.6	870	.01	.02	.1	36
155	Peppers, hot, red, without seeds, dried, ground (chili powder); 1 tablespoon	13	50	2	1	9	20	1.2	11,520	.03	.20	1.6	2
	Potatoes: Baked or boiled; 1 medium, 2½-inch diameter (weight raw, about 5 ounces):												
156	Baked in jacket	75	90	3	Trace	21	9	.7	Trace	.10	.04	1.7	20
157	Boiled; peeled before boiling	80	90	3	Trace	21	9	.7	Trace	.11	.04	1.4	20
158	Chips; 10 medium (2-inch diameter)	3	110	1	7	10	6	.4	Trace	.04	.02	.6	2
	French fried:												
159	Frozen, ready to be heated for serving; 10 pieces (2 by ½ by ½ inch)	64	95	2	4	15	4	.8	Trace	.08	.01	1.2	10
160	Ready-to-eat, deep fat for entire process; 10 pieces (2 by ½ by ½ inch)	45	155	2	7	20	9	.7	Trace	.06	.04	1.8	8

¹ Vitamin A based on yellow corn; white corn contains only a trace.

Nutrients in Common Foods in Terms of Household Measures—Continued

Item number	Food	Water	Food energy	Protein	Fat	Total carbohydrate	Calcium	Iron	Vitamin A value	Thiamine	Riboflavin	Niacin	Ascorbic acid
		Percent	Calories	Grams	Grams	Grams	Milligrams	Milligrams	International Units	Milligrams	Milligrams	Milligrams	Milligrams
	VEGETABLES—Con.												
	Potatoes—Con.												
	Mashed; 1 cup:												
161	Milk added	80	145	4	1	30	47	1.0	50	0.17	0.11	0.2	17
162	Milk and butter added	76	230	4	12	28	45	1.0	470	.16	.10	1.6	16
163	Pumpkin, canned; 1 cup	90	75	2	1	18	46	1.6	7,750	.04	.14	1.2	.....
164	Radishes, raw; 4 small	94	10	Trace	Trace	2	15	.4	10	.01	.01	.1	10
165	Sauerkraut, canned, drained solids; 1 cup	91	30	2	Trace	7	54	.8	60	.05	.10	.2	24
	Spinach:												
166	Cooked; 1 cup	91	45	6	1	6	223	3.6	21,200	.14	.36	1.1	54
167	Canned, creamed, strained; 1 ounce	90	10	1	Trace	2	19	.3	750	.01	.03	.1	1
	Squash:												
	Cooked, 1 cup:												
168	Summer, diced	95	35	1	Trace	8	32	.8	550	.08	.15	1.3	23
169	Winter, baked, mashed	86	95	4	1	23	49	1.6	12,690	.10	.31	1.2	14
170	Canned, strained or chopped; 1 ounce	92	10	Trace	Trace	2	7	.1	510	.01	.01	.1	1
	Sweetpotatoes:												
	Baked or boiled; 1 medium, 5 by 2 inches (weight raw, about 6 ounces):												
171	Baked in jacket	64	155	2	1	36	44	1.0	2 8,970	.10	.07	.7	24
172	Boiled in jacket	71	170	2	1	39	47	1.0	2 11,610	.13	.09	.9	25
173	Candied; 1 small, 3½ by 2 inches	60	295	2	6	60	65	1.6	2 11,030	.10	.08	.8	17
174	Canned, vacuum or solid pack; 1 cup	72	235	4	Trace	54	54	1.7	17,110	.12	.09	1.1	30
	Tomatoes:												
175	Raw; 1 medium (2 by 2½ inches), about ⅓ pound	94	30	2	Trace	6	16	.9	1,640	.08	.06	.8	35
176	Canned or cooked; 1 cup	94	45	2	Trace	9	27	1.5	2,540	.14	.08	1.7	40
177	Tomato juice, canned; 1 cup	94	50	2	Trace	10	17	1.0	2,540	.12	.07	1.8	38
178	Tomato catsup; 1 tablespoon	70	15	Trace	Trace	4	2	.1	320	.02	.01	.4	2

FRUITS

No.	Food												
179	Turnips, cooked, diced; 1 cup	92	40	1	Trace	9	62	.8	Trace	.06	.09	.6	28
180	Turnip greens, cooked; 1 cup	90	45	4	1	8	376	3.5	15,370	.09	.59	1.0	87
181	Apples, raw; 1 medium (2½ inch diameter), about ⅓ pound	85	70	Trace	Trace	18	8	.4	50	.04	.02	.1	3
182	Apple betty; 1 cup	64	350	4	8	69	41	1.4	270	.13	.10	.9	Trace
183	Apple juice, fresh or canned; 1 cup	86	125	Trace	0	34	15	1.2	90	.05	.07	Trace	2
	Apple sauce, canned:												
184	Sweetened; 1 cup	80	185	Trace	Trace	50	10	1.0	80	.05	.03	.1	3
185	Unsweetened; 1 cup	88	100	Trace	Trace	26	10	1.0	70	.05	.02	.1	3
186	Apricots, raw; 3 apricots (about ¼ pound)	85	55	1	Trace	14	18	.5	2,890	.03	.04	.7	10
	Apricots, canned:												
187	Heavy sirup pack, halves and sirup; 1 cup	78	200	1	Trace	54	34	1.0	4,070	.05	.07	1.1	10
188	Water pack, halves and liquid; 1 cup	90	80	1	Trace	21	27	.7	3,320	.04	.05	.9	8
	Apricots, dried:												
189	Uncooked; 1 cup (40 halves, small)	25	390	8	1	100	100	8.2	16,390	.02	.24	4.9	19
190	Cooked unsweetened, fruit and liquid; 1 cup	76	240	5	1	62	63	5.1	10,130	.01	.13	2.8	8
191	Apricots and applesauce, canned, strained or chopped; 1 ounce	80	20	Trace	Trace	5	3	.2	440	.01	.01	.1	Trace
192	Apricot nectar; 1 cup	85	135	1	Trace	36	22	.5	2,380	.02	.02	.5	7
	Avocados, raw, California varieties (mainly Fuerte):												
193	1 cup (½-inch cubes)	74	260	3	26	9	15	.9	430	.16	.30	2.4	21
194	½ of a 10-ounce avocado (3½ by 3¾ inches)	74	185	2	18	6	11	.6	310	.12	.21	1.7	15
	Avocados, raw, Florida varieties:												
195	1 cup (½ inch cubes)	78	195	2	17	13	15	.9	430	.16	.30	2.4	21
196	½ of a 13-ounce avocado (4 by 3 inches)	78	160	2	14	11	12	.7	350	.13	.24	2.0	17
197	Bananas, raw; 1 medium (6 by 1½ inches), about ⅓ pound	76	85	1	Trace	23	10	.7	170	.05	.06	.7	10
198	Blackberries, raw; 1 cup	85	80	2	1	18	46	1.3	280	.05	.06	.5	30
199	Blueberries, raw; 1 cup	83	85	1	1	21	22	1.1	400	.04	.03	.4	23

2 Average vitamin A value for important commercial varieties. Varieties with pale flesh contain very small amounts while those with deep orange-colored flesh have much higher contents than the value shown in the table.

Nutrients in Common Foods in Terms of Household Measures—Continued

Item number	Food	Water (Per cent)	Food energy (Calories)	Protein (Grams)	Fat (Grams)	Total carbohydrate (Grams)	Calcium (Milligrams)	Iron (Milligrams)	Vitamin A value (International Units)	Thiamine (Milligrams)	Riboflavin (Milligrams)	Niacin (Milligrams)	Ascorbic acid (Milligrams)
	FRUITS—Con.												
200	Cantaloupes, raw; ½ melon (5-inch diameter)	94	40	1	Trace	9	33	0.8	[3] 6,590	0.09	0.07	1.0	63
201	Cherries, sour, sweet, and hybrid, raw; 1 cup	83	65	1	1	15	19	.4	650	.05	.06	.4	9
	Cherries, canned:												
202	Red sour, pitted; 1 cup	87	120	2	1	30	28	.8	1,840	.07	.04	.4	14
203	Cranberry juice cocktail, canned; 1 cup	85	135	Trace	Trace	36	10	.5	20	.02	.02	.1	5
204	Cranberry sauce, sweetened; 1 cup	48	550	Trace	Trace	142	22	.8	80	.06	.06	.3	5
205	Dates, "fresh" and dried, pitted and cut; 1 cup	20	505	4	1	134	103	5.3	170	.16	.17	3.9	0
	Figs:												
206	Raw; 3 small (1½-inch diameter), about ¼ pound	78	90	2	Trace	22	62	.7	90	.06	.06	.6	2
207	Dried; 1 large (2 by 1 inch)	23	60	1	Trace	15	43	.3	20	.02	.02	.2	0
208	Fruit cocktail, canned in heavy sirup, solids and liquid; 1 cup	81	175	1	Trace	47	23	1.0	360	.04	.03	1.1	5
	Grapefruit: Raw; ½ medium (4¼-inch diameter, No. 64's):												
209	White	89	50	1	Trace	14	21	.5	10	.05	.02	.2	50
210	Pink or red	89	55	1	Trace	14	21	.5	590	.05	.02	.2	48
211	Raw, sections, white; 1 cup	89	75	1	Trace	20	31	.8	20	.07	.03	.3	72
	Canned:												
212	Sirup pack, solids and liquid; 1 cup	81	165	1	Trace	44	32	.7	20	.07	.04	.5	75
213	Water pack, solids and liquid; 1 cup	91	70	1	Trace	18	31	.7	20	.07	.04	.5	72
	Grapefruit juice:												
214	Raw; 1 cup	90	85	1	Trace	23	22	.5	[4] 20	.09	.04	.4	92
	Canned:												
215	Unsweetened; 1 cup	89	95	1	Trace	24	20	1.0	20	.07	.04	.4	84
216	Sweetened; 1 cup	86	120	1	Trace	32	20	1.0	20	.07	.04	.4	78

No.	Food											
	Frozen concentrate, unsweetened:											
217	Undiluted; 1 can (6 fluid ounces)	62	280	4	1	72	70	.8	60	.29	.12	1.4	286
218	Diluted, ready-to-serve; 1 cup	89	95	1	Trace	24	25	.2	20	.10	.04	.5	96
	Frozen concentrate, sweetened:											
219	Undiluted; 1 can (6 fluid ounces)	57	320	3	1	85	59	.6	50	.24	.11	1.2	245
220	Diluted, ready-to-serve; 1 cup	88	105	1	Trace	28	20	.2	20	.08	.03	.4	82
	Dehydrated:											
221	Crystals; 1 can (net weight 4 ounces)	1	400	5	1	103	99	1.1	90	.41	.18	2.0	399
222	With water added, ready-to-serve; 1 cup	90	90	1	Trace	24	22	.2	20	.10	.05	.5	92
	Grapes, raw; 1 cup:											
223	American type (slip skin)	82	70	1	1	16	13	.4	100	.05	.03	.3	4
224	European type (adherent skin)	81	100	1	Trace	26	18	.6	150	.08	.04	.4	7
225	Grape juice, bottled; 1 cup	82	165	1	1	42	25	.8		.11	.06	.7	Trace
	Lemon juice:											
226	Raw; 1 cup	91	60	1	Trace	20	27	.5	Trace	.08	.03	.3	129
227	Canned; 1 cup	91	60	1	Trace	20	27	.5	Trace	.07	.03	.3	102
	Lemonade concentrate, frozen, sweetened:											
228	Undiluted; 1 can (6 fluid ounces)	48	305	1	Trace	113	9	.4	Trace	.05	.06	.7	67
229	Diluted, ready-to-serve; 1 cup	88	75	Trace	Trace	28	2	.1	Trace	.01	.01	.2	17
	Lime juice:											
230	Raw; 1 cup	90	65	1	Trace	22	22	1.5	Trace	.03	.04	.4	80
231	Canned; 1 cup	90	65	1	Trace	22	22	1.5	Trace	.02	.04	.4	52
	Limeade concentrate, frozen, sweetened:											
232	Undiluted; 1 can (6 fluid ounces)	50	295	Trace	Trace	109	11	.7	Trace	.01	.02	.2	262
233	Diluted, ready-to-serve; 1 cup	90	75	Trace	Trace	27	2	.2	Trace	Trace	.01	.1	6
	Oranges, raw; 1 large orange (3-inch diameter):											
234	Navel	86	70	2	Trace	17	48	.3	270	.11	.03	.4	83
235	Other varieties	86	70	1	Trace	18	63	.3	290	.12	.03	.4	66
	Orange juice:											
	Raw; 1 cup:											
236	California (Valencias)	88	105	2	Trace	26	37	.5	500	.20	.05	.6	126
	Florida varieties:											
237	Early and midseason	90	90	1	Trace	23	25	.5	490	.20	.05	.6	127
238	Late season (Valencias)	88	105	1	Trace	26	25	.5	500	.20	.05	.6	92
239	Canned, unsweetened; 1 cup	87	110	2	Trace	28	25	1.0	500	.17	.05	.6	100

3 Vitamin A based on deeply colored varieties.
4 Vitamin A value for juice from white grapefruit. The vitamin A value per cup of juice from pink or red grapefruit is 1,080 I.U.

Nutrients in Common Foods in Terms of Household Measures—Continued

Item number	Food	Water	Food energy	Protein	Fat	Total carbohydrate	Calcium	Iron	Vitamin A value	Thiamine	Riboflavin	Niacin	Ascorbic acid
		Percent	Calories	Grams	Grams	Grams	Milligrams	Milligrams	International Units	Milligrams	Milligrams	Milligrams	Milligrams
	FRUITS—Con.												
	Orange juice—Con.												
	Frozen concentrate:												
240	Undiluted; 1 can (6 fl. ounces)	58	305	5	Trace	80	69	0.8	1,490	0.63	0.10	2.4	332
241	Diluted, ready-to-serve; 1 cup	88	105	2	Trace	27	22	.2	500	.21	.03	.8	112
	Dehydrated:												
242	Crystals; 1 can (net weight 4 ounces)	1	395	6	2	100	95	1.9	1,900	.76	.19	2.5	406
243	With water added, ready-to-serve; 1 cup	88	105	1	Trace	27	25	.5	500	.20	.05	.6	108
	Orange and grapefruit juice, frozen concentrate:												
244	Undiluted; 1 can (6 fluid ounces)	59	300	4	1	78	61	.8	790	.47	.06	2.3	301
245	Diluted, ready-to-serve; 1 cup	88	100	1	Trace	26	20	.2	270	.16	.02	.8	102
	Peaches:												
	Raw:												
246	1 medium (2½ by 2-inch diameter), about ¼ pound	89	35	1	Trace	10	9	.5	[5]1,320	.02	.05	1.0	7
247	1 cup, sliced	89	65	1	Trace	16	15	.8	[5]2,230	.03	.08	1.6	12
	Canned (yellow-fleshed) solids and liquid:												
248	Heavy-sirup pack; 1 cup	80	185	1	Trace	49	13	.8	1,000	.02	.06	1.3	8
249	Water pack; 1 cup	92	65	1	Trace	17	15	.7	1,100	.02	.07	1.4	9
250	Strained; 1 ounce	82	20	Trace	Trace	5	2	.2	150	Trace	.01	.2	Trace
	Dried:												
251	Uncooked; 1 cup	25	420	5	1	109	80	9.6	6,330	.02	.32	8.4	32
252	Cooked, unsweetened; 1 cup (10-12 halves and 6 tablespoons liquid)	77	220	3	1	58	43	5.1	3,350	.01	.16	4.1	6
	Frozen:												
253	1 12-ounce carton	79	265	1	Trace	69	20	1.4	1,770	.04	.10	1.8	[6]99
254	1 16-ounce can	79	355	2	Trace	92	27	1.8	2,360	.05	.14	2.4	[6]132
255	Peach nectar, canned; 1 cup	87	115	Trace	Trace	31	10	.5	1,070	.02	.05	1.0	1

No.	Food												
	Pears:												
256	Raw; 1 pear (3- by 2½-inch diameter)........	83	100	1	1	25	13	.5	30	.04	.07	.2	7
	Canned, solids and liquid:												
257	Heavy-sirup pack; 1 cup........	81	175	1	Trace	47	18	1.3	10	.02	.05	.4	3
258	Strained; 1 ounce.............	84	15	Trace	Trace	4	3	.1	Trace	Trace	.01	.1	Trace
259	Pear nectar, canned; 1 cup......	86	125	1	Trace	33	8	.2	10	.01	.05	Trace	1
	Pineapple:												
260	Raw, diced; 1 cup.............	85	75	1	Trace	19	22	.4	180	.12	.04	.3	33
	Canned:												
	Sirup pack, solids and liquid:												
261	Crushed; 1 cup............	78	205	1	Trace	55	75	1.6	210	.20	.04	.4	23
262	Sliced; 2 small or 1 large slice and 2 tablespoons juice....	78	95	Trace	Trace	26	35	.7	100	.09	.02	.2	11
263	Pineapple juice, canned; 1 cup..	86	120	Trace	Trace	32	37	1.2	200	.13	.04	.4	22
	Plums:												
264	Raw; 1 plum (2-inch diameter), about 2 ounces........	86	30	Trace	Trace	7	10	.3	200	.04	.02	.3	3
	Canned (Italian prunes):												
265	Sirup pack, solids and liquid; 1 cup....	79	185	1	Trace	50	20	2.7	560	.07	.06	.9	3
	Prunes, dried:												
266	Uncooked; 4 medium prunes....	24	70	1	Trace	19	14	1.0	430	.02	.05	.5	1
267	Cooked, unsweetened; 1 cup (17-18 prunes and ⅓ cup liquid)....	65	295	3	1	78	57	4.3	1,780	.08	.18	1.7	3
268	Canned, strained; 1 ounce....	73	25	Trace	Trace	7	8	.4	170	.01	.01	.2	1
269	Prune juice, canned; 1 cup....	80	170	1	Trace	45	36	10.6	......	.01	.03	1.1	4
270	Raisins, dried; 1 cup......	18	460	4	Trace	124	99	6.2	30	.13	.12	.7	2
	Raspberries, red:												
271	Raw; 1 cup............	84	70	1	Trace	17	49	1.1	160	.03	.08	.4	29
272	Frozen; 10-ounce carton....	74	280	2	1	70	79	1.7	220	.03	.12	.5	45
273	Rhubarb, cooked, sugar added; 1 cup..	63	385	1	Trace	98	112	1.1	70	.02	......	.2	17
	Strawberries:												
274	Raw; 1 cup.......	90	55	1	1	12	42	1.2	90	.04	.10	.4	89
275	Frozen; 10-ounce carton....	72	300	2	1	75	62	1.7	120	.05	.14	.5	116
276	Frozen; 16-ounce can....	72	485	3	2	121	100	2.7	190	.08	.23	.8	186
277	Tangerines; 1 medium (2½-inch diameter), about ¼ pound....	87	40	1	Trace	10	34	.3	360	.05	.01	.1	26

[5] Vitamin A value of yellow-fleshed varieties; the value is negligible in white-fleshed varieties.
[6] Content of frozen peaches with added ascorbic acid; when not added the content is 14 milligrams per 12-ounce carton and 18 milligrams per 16-ounce can.

Nutrients in Common Foods in Terms of Household Measures—Continued

Item number	Food	Water	Food energy	Protein	Fat	Total carbohydrate	Calcium	Iron	Vitamin A value	Thiamine	Riboflavin	Niacin	Ascorbic acid
		Percent	Calories	Grams	Grams	Grams	Milligrams	Milligrams	International Units	Milligrams	Milligrams	Milligrams	Milligrams
	FRUITS—Con.												
	Tangerine juice:												
278	Canned; 1 cup............	89	100	1	Trace	25	45	0.5	1,050	0.14	0.04	0.3	56
	Frozen concentrate:												
279	Undiluted; 6-fluid-ounce can...	58	315	4	1	80	130	1.5	3,070	.43	.12	.9	202
280	Diluted, ready-to-serve; 1 cup. .	88	105	1	Trace	27	45	.5	1,020	.14	.04	.3	67
281	Watermelon; 1 wedge (4 by 8 inches), about 2 pounds (weighed with rind)..	92	120	2	1	29	30	.9	2,530	.20	.22	.7	26
	GRAIN PRODUCTS												
282	Biscuits, baking powder, enriched flour; 1 biscuit (2½-inch diameter)...	27	130	3	4	20	83	.7	0	.09	.08	.7	0
283	Bran flakes (40 percent bran) with added thiamine; 1 ounce...	4	85	3	1	22	17	1.1	0	.13	.07	2.5	0
	Breads:												
	Cracked wheat:												
284	1 pound (20 slices)........	35	1,190	39	10	236	399	5.0	Trace	.53	.42	5.8	Trace
285	1 slice (½ inch thick).......	35	60	2	1	12	20	.3	Trace	.03	.02	.3	Trace
	French or vienna:												
286	Enriched; 1 pound.........	31	1,315	41	14	251	195	10.0	Trace	1.26	.98	11.3	Trace
287	Unenriched; 1 pound.......	31	1,315	41	14	251	195	3.2	Trace	.39	.39	3.6	Trace
	Italian:												
288	Enriched; 1 pound.........	32	1,250	41	4	256	77	10.0	0	1.31	.93	11.7	0
289	Unenriched; 1 pound.......	32	1,250	41	4	256	77	3.2	0	.39	.27	3.6	0
	Raisin:												
290	1 pound (20 slices)........	35	1,190	30	13	243	322	5.9	Trace	.24	.42	3.0	Trace
291	1 slice (½ inch thick).... ..	35	60	2	1	12	16	.3	Trace	.01	.02	.2	Trace
	Rye:												
	American (light):												
292	1 pound (20 slices)........	36	1,100	41	5	236	340	7.3	0	.81	.33	6.4	0
293	1 slice (½ inch thick)......	36	55	2	Trace	12	17	.4	0	.04	.02	.3	0
	Pumpernickel:												
294	1 pound..................	34	1,115	41	5	241	381	10.9	0	1.05	.63	5.4	0

Item	Food												
	White:[7]												
	Enriched, made with—												
	1-2 percent nonfat dry milk:												
295	1 pound (20 slices)........	36	1,225	39	15	229	318	10.9	Trace	1.13	.77	10.4	Trace
296	1 slice (½ inch thick)........	36	60	2	1	12	16	.6	Trace	.06	.04	.5	Trace
	3-4 percent nonfat dry milk:												
297	1 pound (20 slices)........	36	1,225	39	15	229	381	11.3	Trace	1.13	.95	10.8	Trace
298	1 slice (½ inch thick)........	36	60	2	1	12	19	.6	Trace	.06	.05	.6	Trace
	5-6 percent nonfat dry milk:												
299	1 pound (20 slices)........	35	1,245	41	17	228	435	11.3	Trace	1.22	.91	11.0	Trace
300	1 slice (½ inch thick)........	35	65	2	1	12	22	.6	Trace	.06	.05	.6	Trace
	Unenriched, made with—												
	1-2 percent nonfat dry milk:												
301	1 pound (20 slices)........	36	1,225	39	15	229	318	3.2	Trace	.40	.36	5.6	Trace
302	1 slice (½ inch thick)........	36	60	2	1	12	16	.2	Trace	.02	.02	.3	Trace
	3-4 percent nonfat dry milk:												
303	1 pound (20 slices)........	36	1,225	39	15	229	381	3.2	Trace	.31	.39	5.0	Trace
304	1 slice (½ inch thick)........	36	60	2	1	12	19	.2	Trace	.02	.02	.3	Trace
	5-6 percent nonfat dry milk:												
305	1 pound (20 slices)........	35	1,245	41	17	228	435	3.2	Trace	.32	.59	4.1	Trace
306	1 slice (½ inch thick)........	35	65	2	1	12	22	.2	Trace	.02	.03	.2	Trace
	Whole wheat, graham, or entire wheat:												
307	1 pound (20 slices)........	36	1,105	48	14	216	449	10.4	Trace	1.17	1.03	12.9	Trace
308	1 slice (½ inch thick)........	36	55	2	1	11	23	.5	Trace	.06	.05	.7	Trace
	Cakes:												
309	Angelfood; 2-inch sector (1/12 of cake, 8-inch diameter)........	32	110	3	Trace	23	2	.1	0	Trace	.05	.1	0
	Butter cakes:												
	Plain cake and cupcakes without icing:												
310	1 square (3 by 2 by 1½ inches)........	27	180	4	5	31	85	.2	70[8]	.02	.05	.2	0
311	1 cupcake (2¾-inch diameter)........	27	130	3	3	23	62	.2	50[8]	.01	.03	.1	0
	Plain cake with icing:												
312	2-inch sector of iced layer cake (1/16 of cake, 10-inch diameter)........	25	320	5	6	62	117	.4	90[8]	.02	.07	.2	0

[7] When the amount of nonfat dry milk in commercial bread is unknown, use bread with 3-4 percent nonfat dry milk.

[8] If the fat used in the recipe were butter or fortified margarine, the vitamin A value for plain cake would be 200 I.U. per large square, item 310; 150 I.U. per cupcake, item 311; 280 I.U. per 2-inch sector, iced, item 312; for rich cake, 900 I.U. per 2-inch sector, iced, item 313; for fruit cake 120 I.U. per piece (2 by 2 by ½ inches), item 314.

Nutrients in Common Foods in Terms of Household Measures—Continued

Item number	Food	Water	Food energy	Protein	Fat	Total carbohydrate	Calcium	Iron	Vitamin A value	Thiamine	Riboflavin	Niacin	Ascorbic acid
		Percent	Calories	Grams	Grams	Grams	Milligrams	Milligrams	International Units	Milligrams	Milligrams	Milligrams	Milligrams
	GRAIN PRODUCTS—Con.												
	Cakes—Con.												
	Butter cakes—Con.												
	Rich cake:												
313	2-inch sector of layer cake, iced (1/16 of cake, 10-inch diameter)	21	490	6	19	76	114	0.6	[8] 220	0.03	0.10	0.2	0
314	Fruit cake, dark; 1 piece (2 by 2 by 1/2 inches)	23	105	2	4	17	29	.8	[8] 50	.04	.04	.3	0
315	Gingerbread; 1 piece (2 by 2 by 2 inches)	30	180	2	7	28	63	1.4	50	.02	.05	.6	0
316	Sponge; 2-inch sector (1/12 of cake, 8-inch diameter)	32	115	3	2	22	11	.6	210	.02	.06	.1	0
317	Cookies, plain and assorted; 1 cookie (3-inch diameter)	5	110	2	3	19	6	.2	0	.01	.01	.1	0
318	Cornbread or muffins made with enriched, degermed cornmeal; 1 muffin (2¾-inch diameter)	49	105	3	2	18	67	.9	[9] 60	.08	.11	.6	0
319	Corn, puffed, presweetened, added thiamine, riboflavin, niacin, and iron; 1 ounce	3	110	1	Trace	26	3	.5	....	.12	.05	.5	0
320	Corn and soy shreds, added thiamine and niacin; 1 ounce	4	100	5	Trace	21	24	1.2	....	.19	.04	.6	0
321	Corn cereal mixture (mainly degermed cornmeal) puffed, added thiamine, niacin, and iron; 1 ounce	3	115	2	1	23	6	1.2	....	.15	.04	.6	0
	Cornflakes:												
322	With added thiamine, niacin, and iron; 1 ounce	4	110	2	Trace	24	3	.5	0	.12	.03	.6	0
323	Presweetened, added thiamine, niacin, and iron; 1 ounce	4	110	1	Trace	26	1	.5	0	.12	.01	.6	0
	Corn grits, degermed, cooked:												
324	Enriched; 1 cup	87	120	3	Trace	27	2	.7	[10] 100	.11	.08	1.0	0

No.	Food												
325	Unenriched; 1 cup............	87	120	3	Trace	27	2	.2	[10] 100	.04	.01	.4	0
	Crackers:												
326	Graham; 4 small or 2 medium......	6	55	1	1	10	3	.3	0	.04	.02	.2	0
327	Saltines; 2 crackers (2-inch square).	5	35	1	1	6	2	.1	0	Trace	Trace	.1	0
	Soda, plain:												
328	2 crackers (2½-inch square).....	6	45	1	1	8	2	.1	0	.01	.01	.1	0
329	10 oyster crackers or 1 tablespoon cracker meal......	6	45	1	1	7	2	.1	0	.01	Trace	.1	0
330	Doughnuts, cake type; 1 doughnut....	19	135	2	7	17	23	.4	40	.05	.04	.4	0
331	Farina, enriched to minimum levels for required nutrients and for the optional nutrient, calcium; cooked; 1 cup.....	89	105	3	Trace	22	31	.8	0	.11	.07	1.0	0
	Macaroni, cooked; 1 cup: Enriched:												
332	Cooked 8-10 minutes (undergoes additional cooking as ingredient of a food mixture)......	64	190	6	1	39	14	1.4	0	.23	.14	1.9	0
333	Cooked until tender..........	72	155	5	1	32	11	1.3	0	.19	.11	1.5	0
	Unenriched:												
334	Cooked 8-10 minutes (undergoes additional cooking as ingredient of a food mixture).....	64	190	6	1	39	14	.6	0	.02	.02	.5	0
335	Cooked until tender..........	72	155	5	1	32	11	.6	0	.02	.02	.4	0
336	Macaroni and cheese, baked (enriched macaroni used); 1 cup.....	58	475	18	25	44	394	2.0	970	.22	.46	1.9	Trace
337	Muffins, made with enriched white flour; 1 muffin (2¾-inch diameter)......	37	135	4	4	20	99	.8	50	.09	.10	.7	0
	Noodles (egg noodles), cooked:												
338	Enriched; 1 cup...........	70	200	7	2	37	16	1.4	60	.23	.14	1.8	0
339	Unenriched; 1 cup..........	70	200	7	2	37	16	1.0	60	.04	.03	.7	0
340	Oat cereal (mixture, mainly oat flour), ready-to-eat, added B vitamins and minerals; 1 ounce.........	3	115	4	2	21	45	1.2	0	.22	.04	.5	0
341	Oatmeal or rolled oats, regular or quick cooking, cooked; 1 cup...	85	150	5	3	26	21	1.7	0	.22	.05	.4	0

[9] Based on recipe using white cornmeal; if yellow cornmeal is used vitamin A value is 120 I.U.
[10] Vitamin A based on yellow corn grits; white corn grits contain only a trace.

Nutrients in Common Foods in Terms of Household Measures—Continued

Item number	Food	Water	Food energy	Protein	Fat	Total carbohydrate	Calcium	Iron	Vitamin A value	Thiamine	Riboflavin	Niacin	Ascorbic acid
		Percent	Calories	Grams	Grams	Grams	Milligrams	Milligrams	International Units	Milligrams	Milligrams	Milligrams	Milligrams
	GRAIN PRODUCTS—Con.												
	Pancakes, baked; 1 cake (4-inch diameter):												
342	Wheat (home recipe)	55	60	2	2	7	43	0.2	50	0.02	0.03	0.1	Trace
343	Buckwheat (with buckwheat pancake mix)	62	45	2	2	6	67	.3	30	.04	.04	.2	Trace
	Pies; 4-inch sector (1/7 of 9-inch diameter pie):												
344	Apple	48	330	3	13	53	9	.5	220	.04	.02	.3	1
345	Cherry	46	340	3	13	55	14	.5	520	.04	.02	.3	2
346	Custard	58	265	7	11	34	162	1.6	290	.07	.21	.4	0
347	Lemon meringue	47	300	4	12	45	24	.6	210	.04	.10	.2	1
348	Mince	43	340	3	9	62	22	3.0	10	.09	.05	.5	1
349	Pumpkin	59	265	5	12	34	70	1.0	2,480	.04	.15	.4	0
350	Pretzels; 5 small sticks	8	20	Trace	Trace	4	1	.0	0	Trace	Trace	Trace	0
	Rice, cooked; 1 cup:												
351	Converted	72	205	4	Trace	45	14	.5	0	.10	.02	1.9	0
352	White	71	200	4	Trace	44	13	.5	0	.02	.01	.7	0
353	Rice, puffed, added thiamine, niacin, and iron; 1 ounce	5	110	2	Trace	25	4	.5	0	.12	.01	1.5	0
354	Rice flakes, added thiamine and niacin; 1 ounce	5	110	2	Trace	25	8	.6	0	.10	.01	1.6	0
	Rolls:												
	Plain, pan (16 ounces per dozen); 1 roll:												
355	Enriched	31	115	3	2	20	28	.7	Trace	.11	.07	.8	Trace
356	Unenriched	31	115	3	2	20	28	.3	Trace	.02	.03	.3	Trace
357	Hard, round (22 ounces per dozen); 1 roll	25	160	5	2	31	24	.4	Trace	.03	.05	.4	Trace
358	Sweet, pan (18 ounces per dozen); 1 roll	31	135	4	4	21	37	.3	30	.03	.06	.4	0
359	Spaghetti, cooked until tender: Enriched; 1 cup	72	155	5	1	32	11	1.3	0	.19	.11	1.5	0

No.	Food	Grams	Calories	Protein (g)	Fat (g)	Carbohydrate (g)	Calcium (mg)	Iron (mg)	Vitamin A (I.U.)	Thiamine (mg)	Riboflavin (mg)	Niacin (mg)	Ascorbic acid (mg)
360	Unenriched; 1 cup	72	155	5	1	32	11	.6	0	.02	.02	.4	0
	Waffles, baked, with enriched flour:												
361	1 waffle (4½ by 5½ by ½ inches)	40	215	7	8	28	144	1.4	270	.14	.20	1.0	0
	Wheat, puffed:												
362	Added thiamine, niacin, and iron; 1 ounce	4	100	4	Trace	22	8	1.2	0	.16	.06	2.2	0
363	Presweetened, added thiamine and niacin; 1 ounce	3	105	1	Trace	26	4	.5	0	.12	.01	1.4	0
364	Wheat, rolled, cooked; 1 cup	80	175	5	1	40	19	1.7	0	.17	.06	2.1	0
365	Wheat, shredded, plain (long, round, or bite-size); 1 ounce	6	100	3	1	23	13	1.0	0	.06	.03	1.3	0
366	Wheat and malted barley cereal, added thiamine, niacin, and iron; 1 ounce	3	105	3	Trace	24	13	1.0	0	.13	.05	1.5	0
367	Wheat flakes, added thiamine, niacin, and iron; 1 ounce	4	100	3	Trace	23	13	1.2	0	.16	.05	1.8	0
	Wheat flours:												
368	Whole wheat; 1 cup, stirred	12	400	16	2	85	49	4.0	0	.66	.14	5.2	0
	All purpose or family flour:												
369	Enriched; 1 cup, sifted	12	400	12	1	84	18	[11]3.2	0	[11].48	[11].29	[11]3.8	0
370	Unenriched; 1 cup, sifted	12	400	12	1	84	18	.9	0	.07	.05	1.0	0
371	Wheat germ; 1 cup, stirred	11	245	17	7	34	57	5.5	0	1.39	.54	3.1	0

FATS, OILS, RELATED PRODUCTS

No.	Food	Grams	Calories	Protein (g)	Fat (g)	Carbohydrate (g)	Calcium (mg)	Iron (mg)	Vitamin A (I.U.)	Thiamine (mg)	Riboflavin (mg)	Niacin (mg)	Ascorbic acid (mg)
372	Butter; 1 tablespoon	14	100	Trace	11	Trace	3	0	[12]460	......	......	......	0
	Fats, cooking:												
	Vegetable fats:												
373	1 cup	200	1,770	0	200	0	0	0	0	0	0	0	0
374	1 tablespoon	12	110	0	12	0	0	0	0	0	0	0	0
	Lard:												
375	1 cup	220	1,985	0	220	0	0	0	0	0	0	0	0
376	1 tablespoon	14	125	0	14	Trace	0	0	0	0	0	0	0
377	Margarine; 1 tablespoon	14	100	Trace	11	Trace	3	0	[13]460	0	0	......	0
378	Oils, salad or cooking; 1 tablespoon	14	125	0	14	0	0	0	0	0	0	0	0

[11] Iron, thiamine, riboflavin, and niacin are based on the minimal level of enrichment specified in the standards of identity promulgated under the Federal Food, Drug, and Cosmetic Act.

[12] Year-round average.

[13] Based on the average vitamin A content of fortified margarine. Federal specifications for fortified margarine require a minimum of 15,000 I.U. of vitamin A per pound.

Nutrients in Common Foods in Terms of Household Measures—Continued

Item number	Food	Water	Food energy	Protein	Fat	Total carbohydrate	Calcium	Iron	Vitamin A value	Thiamine	Riboflavin	Niacin	Ascorbic acid
		Percent	Calories	Grams	Grams	Grams	Milligrams	Milligrams	International Units	Milligrams	Milligrams	Milligrams	Milligrams
	FATS, OILS, RELATED PRODUCTS—Continued												
	Salad dressings; 1 tablespoon:												
379	Blue cheese	28	90	1	10	1	11	Trace	30	Trace	0.02	Trace	Trace
380	Commercial, plain (mayonnaise type)	48	60	Trace	6	2	2	Trace	30	Trace	Trace	Trace	0
381	French	42	60	Trace	6	2	3	.1	0	0	0	0	0
382	Mayonnaise	14	110	Trace	12	Trace	2	.1	40	Trace	Trace	Trace	0
383	Thousand Island	38	75	Trace	8	1	2	.1	60	Trace	Trace	Trace	2
	SUGARS, SWEETS												
	Candy; 1 ounce:												
384	Caramels	7	120	1	3	22	36	.7	50	.01	.04	Trace	Trace
385	Chocolate, sweetened, milk	1	145	2	9	16	61	.3	40	.03	.11	.2	0
386	Fudge, plain	5	115	Trace	3	23	14	.1	60	Trace	.02	Trace	Trace
387	Hard	1	110	0	0	28	0	0	0	0	0	0	0
388	Marshmallow	15	90	1	0	23	0	0	0	0	0	0	0
389	Chocolate sirup; 1 tablespoon	39	40	Trace	Trace	11	3	.3	.....	.....	.....	.....	.....
390	Honey, strained or extracted; 1 tablespoon	20	60	Trace	0	17	1	.2	0	Trace	.01	Trace	1
391	Jams, marmalades, preserves; 1 tablespoon	28	55	Trace	Trace	14	2	.1	Trace	Trace	Trace	Trace	1
392	Jellies; 1 tablespoon	34	50	0	0	13	2	.1	Trace	Trace	Trace	Trace	1
	Molasses, cane; 1 tablespoon:												
393	Light	24	50	.....	.....	13	33	.9	.....	.01	.01	Trace	.....
394	Blackstrap	24	45	.....	.....	11	116	2.3	.....	.02	.04	.3	.....
395	Sirup, table blends; 1 tablespoon	25	55	0	0	15	3	.8	0	0	Trace	Trace	0
	Sugar; 1 tablespoon:												
396	Granulated, cane or beet	Trace	50	0	0	12	.....	.....	0	0	0	0	0
397	Brown	3	50	0	0	13	[14]10	.4	0	0	0	0	0

MISCELLANEOUS

398	Beverages, carbonated, cola type; 1 cup	88	105	Trace	Trace	28	……	……	……	……	.07	1.0	0
399	Bouillon cubes; 1 cube	5	2	Trace	Trace	0	……	……	……	……	……	……	……
400	Chili sauce (mainly tomatoes); 1 tablespoon	69	15	Trace	Trace	4	2	.1	320	.02	.01	.4	2
401	Chocolate, unsweetened; 1 ounce	2	145	2	15	8	28	1.2	20	.01	.06	.3	0
402	Gelatin dessert, plain, ready-to-serve; 1 cup	83	155	4	0	36	0	0	0	0	0	0	0
	Olives, pickled; "Extra large" size, 12 olives or "Jumbo" size, 7 olives:												
403	Green	78	65	1	7	1	48	.9	170	Trace	Trace	……	……
404	Ripe	76	85	1	9	2	45	.9	40	Trace	Trace	……	……
	Pickles, cucumber:												
405	Dill; 1 large (4 inches long, 1¾-inch diameter)	93	15	1	Trace	3	34	1.6	420	Trace	.09	.1	8
406	Sweet; 1 pickle (2¾ inches long, ¾-inch diameter)	70	20	Trace	Trace	5	3	.3	20	0	Trace	Trace	1
407	Sherbet, factory packed; 1 cup (8-fluid-ounce container)	68	235	3	3	58	96	.1	0	.03	.15	.1	0
	Soups, ready-to-serve; 1 cup:												
408	Bean	82	190	8	5	30	95	2.8	……	.10	.10	.8	……
409	Beef	92	100	6	4	11	15	1.5	0	……	……	……	0
410	Bouillon, broth, and consomme	95	10	2	……	0	2	1.0	……	0	.05	.6	……
411	Chicken	94	75	4	2	10	20	.5	……	.02	.12	1.5	……
412	Clam chowder	91	85	5	2	12	36	3.6	……	……	……	……	……
413	Cream soup (asparagus, celery, or mushroom)	85	200	7	12	18	217	.5	200	.05	.20	.1	0
414	Noodle, rice, or barley	90	115	6	4	13	82	.2	30	.02	.05	.7	0
415	Tomato	91	90	2	2	18	24	1.0	1,230	.02	.10	.7	10
416	Vegetable	92	80	4	2	14	32	.8	……	.05	.08	1.0	8
417	Vinegar; 1 tablespoon	……	2	0	……	1	1	.1	……	……	……	……	……
418	White sauce, medium; 1 cup	73	430	10	33	23	305	.3	1,350	.07	.42	.3	1

[14] Calcium value is based on dark brown sugar; value would be lower for light brown sugar.

Following is a food composition table for specialty foods used in this diet. These tables are incomplete in some places because they contain only information furnished by the companies that manufacture the specific products.

	Protein	Carbohydrate	Fat	Calories
Wheat flour 1 c. sifted	11.6	83.7	1.1	400
Cellu Products				
Soybean flour 1 cup	42.1	10.7	23.3	420.9
Rice flour 1 c.	10.7	122.3	0.5	540.5
1 T.	.7	7.6	.03	33.8
Potato starch flour 1 c.	.8	140.9	0.3	569.5
Tapioca flour 1 c.	0.9	131.3	0.3	531.5
1 T.	.18	8.2	.01	33.2
Grainless mix 1 c.	17.9	56.5	21.3	489.3
Nu-Vita				
Puffed brown rice 1 c.	0.8	12.3	0.1	55.0
Puffed millet 1 c.	1.3	–	–	43.0
Ralston-Purina				
Rice Chex 1 c.	1.3	20.8	.08	95.2
Fearn Soya				
Rice baking mix 1 c.	–	117.0	–	493
Jolly Joan				
Rice mix 1 c.	6.9	121.8	.31	518
Potato mix 1 c.	1.55	137.9	.04	500
Rice polish 1 c.	12.8	51.4	13.2	392
El Molino				
Sesame seeds, ½ c.	5.5	50.3	16.0	174.6
Potato flour 1 c.	18	140.9	.3	569.5
1 T.	1.1	8.8	.02	35.6
Syntex Laboratories				
Soy base: Dilute, 2 parts water: 1 part formula 1 c.	4.3	15.4	8.5	155.3
Soy base, Undilute 1 c.	17.2	61.6	34.0	621.2
Knox gelatin, 1 pkg.	7.0	–	–	28
Diet Imperial Margarine 1 t.	–	–	1.8	16.0
1 T.	–	–	5.4	48
Brown sugar 1 T.	–	13	–	50

5

Determining Food Allergens

Food families are important in food allergies because a person who is allergic to one food often finds he cannot eat other foods in the same group. He knows that other foods in the group must be suspect and is very careful in adding them to his diet. Some allergens may be identified only by trial and error. If your child apparently has a reaction to a specific food, eliminate that food from his diet for at least two weeks. Then try it again. If another reaction occurs, you can be fairly sure that the food in question is the culprit. Below is a listing of food families and their components.

BIOLOGICAL CLASSIFICATION OF ANIMALS

MAMMALS

Cow (beef, veal, cow's milk and milk products)
Goat (goat's milk and milk products).
Sheep (mutton, lamb)

Rabbit
Squirrel
Pig (pork, ham, bacon)
Deer (venison)

BIRDS

Chicken
Goose
Turkey
Duck

Pheasant
Guinea Fowl
Cornish game hens
Partridge—Quail

CRUSTACEANS

Salt Water

Crabs
Lobsters
Shrimps

Fresh Water

Crayfish

Biological Classification of Animals (cont.)

Salt Water   *Fresh Water*

MOLLUSKS

Oysters	Clams	Clams
Scallops	Squid	
Abalone		

FISH

Ocean Perch	Bonito	Perch	Crappie
Flounder	Grouper	Whitefish	Pickerel
Cod	Rockfish	Salmon	Grayling
Tuna	Sole	Sunfish	Dru
Swordfish	Red snapper	Carp	Bullhead
Sea bass	Black bass	Pike	Smelt
Eel	Pompano	Bass	Catfish
Herring	Mullet	Sturgeon	Muskellunge
Anchovy	Croaker	Trout—mountain	
Sardine	Weakfish	and lake	
Haddock	White bass	Shad	
Halibut	Redfish		
Mackerel			

BOTANICAL RELATIONSHIP OF EDIBLE PLANTS

*Means not edible but often encountered.

APPLE

Apple
Pectin
Cider
Vinegar
Crabapple
Pear
 Quince (gum)

ALGAE (Gums)

Irish moss (used
in toothpaste
and laxatives)
Agar-agar
Kelp
Carrageen

BANANA

Banana
Plantain

BEECH

Chestnut
Beechnut

BIRCH

Butternut
*Oil of birch
(used in perfume)
Filbert
Hazelnut

BUCKWHEAT

Buckwheat
Rhubarb
Garden sorrel

CAPER

Capers

CASHEWS

Cashews
Pistachio
Mango

*Poison Ivy
*Poison Sumac

CARROTS

Anise
Angelica
Caraway seeds
Carrots
Celery
Coriander
Cumin
Dill
Fennel
Parsley
Parsnips

Botanical Relationship of Edible Plants (cont.)

CEREAL GRAINS

Barley
  Malt
  Oats
Wheat
  Bran
  Graham flour
  Gluten flour
Millet
Corn
  Hominy

Bamboo Shoots
Rice
Wild rice
Sorghum
  Kafir
Cane
  Cane sugar
  Molasses

CITRUS

Bergamot
Citron
Grapefruit
Kumquat
Lemon
Lime
Orange
Tangerine

COLA NUT

Chocolate
Cocoa
Cola (soft drinks)

FUNGI

Mushrooms
Yeast

GINGER

Arrowroot
Cardamon
Ginger
Turmeric
Vanilla

GOOSEBERRY

Black currant
Red currant
Gooseberry

GOOSEFOOT

Spinach
Beets
Sugar beets
Swiss chard

GOURD

Casaba melon
Cantaloupe
Cristman melon
Cucumber
Honeydew
Muskmelon
Persian melon
Pumpkin
Squash
Watermelon

GRAPE

Grapes
Raisins
Cream of tartar
Wine vinegar
Wine
Brandy
Champagne

HEATH

Blueberry
Cranberry
Huckleberry
Wintergreen

LAUREL

Bay leaves
Avocado
*Camphor (used in
  many old remedies)
Cassia
Cinnamon
Sassafras

LEGUMES

Alfalfa
Clover
Carob *or* St. John's
  Bread (gum)
Coffee bean
Black-eyed peas
Peas
Chickpea *or*
garbanzo
Lentil
Stringbean
Lima bean
Soybean
Navy bean
Kidney bean
Jack bean
Tonka bean
Mung bean (used
  to sprout bean
  sprouts)
Peanut
Tamarind
Licorice

Gum Arabic
*Gum Tragacanth
* Senna (artificial
  cinnamon also
  used as laxative)

LILY

Asparagus
Chives
Garlic
Leek
Onion
Shallot
Sarsaparilla

MALLOW

Cottonseed oil
Cottonseed meal
Okra (gumbo)

MINT

Basil
Horehound
Marjoram
Mint
Oregano
Peppermint
Rosemary
Spearmint
Sage
Savory
Thyme

MORNING GLORY

Sweet potato
Yam

Botanical Relationship of Edible Plants (cont.)

MULBERRY

Breadfruit
Fig
Hops
Mulberry

MUSTARD

Cauliflower
Cabbage
Celery cabbage
Chinese cabbage
Colza shoots
Collards
Brussels sprouts
Broccoli
Horseradish
Kohlrabi
Kale
Mustard
Radish
Rutabaga
Turnip
Watercress

MYRTLE

Allspice
Cloves
Guava

NIGHTSHADE

Cayenne pepper
Chili pepper
Red and green
peppers
Eggplant
Potato
*Tobacco
Tomato

NUTMEG

Mace
Nutmeg

PALM

Coconut
Coconut oil
Dates
Palm cabbage
Sago

PEPPER

Black pepper
White pepper
Peppercorns

PINEAPPLE

Pineapple

PLUM

Almond
Apricot
Cherry
Nectarine
Peach
Plum
Prune
Sloe berry (sloe gin)

ROSE

Boysenberry
Dewberry
Loganberry
Blackberry
Black raspberry
Red raspberry
Strawberry
Youngberry

SPURGE

Jassava meal
Tapioca

STERCULA

Chocolate
Cocoa
Cocoa butter
Cola beans

THISTLE

Artichoke
Celtuce
Chicory
Dandelion
Escarole
Endive
Jerusalem
artichoke
Lettuce
Oyster plant
Safflower
Salsify
Sunflower seeds
Tarragon

WALNUT

Hickory
Pecan
Walnut

The foods below all
contain caffeine:

Coffee
Cocoa
**Khat
Tea
Chocolate

**Guarana
Cola
**Cassine
Mate

**See glossary for
definition

A food has mold if it belongs to the following groups:

1. Any food that has been aged in any way
   vinegar
   wine
   corned beef
   cider and homemade root beer
   pickled foods (pickles, relish, pickled beets, catsup) ground meat, unless ground fresh
2. Any smoked foods—however, some are not moldy if they are cooked and packed right away. Check with your meat dealer.
   ham
   sausages
   corned beef
   many delicatessen foods
   frankfurters
   smoked fish
3. Any leftovers that have been kept for more than one day.
4. Melons—especially cantaloupe
5. Mushrooms
6. Soy sauce
7. Canned tomatoes, unless homemade
8. All dried fruits
   raisins
   prunes
   dried apricots
   figs and dates
9. You may also find that grapes and grape juice cause difficulty. They have a natural mold used to make wine.

Knowing what allergens trouble your child is vital to his health. The ten leading causes of allergy have been identified as: cow's milk, chocolate and cola, corn, eggs, legumes (chiefly peanuts), citrus fruits, tomato, wheat, cinnamon, dyes and additives.

Identifying the allergens doesn't help much if you have no substitute for them in your cooking. The following chapter will help you make substitutions so you will be able to utilize some of your family favorites.

6

Reading Labels and Making Substitutions

It is impossible to do a thorough job of eliminating allergens from your child's diet without learning to read labels. For example, the label may say "malt" and if you don't know that this is one form of gluten you're in trouble. It may say dextrose, which is actually a corn product.

Admittedly, label-reading can become very frustrating, but think of the joy of finally finding something that is free of allergens. Think of label-reading as a treasure hunt!

Remember that there are several words that mean the same thing on labels. You can often get a complete list of these ingredients from your doctor or your county health department's dietitian. She can help you formulate your diet and answer some of your questions. When you see any of the words on the following lists on a label it is an indication that the product contains corn, wheat, gluten, egg or citric acid. These should be eliminated from your child's diet.

GLUTEN

Wheat—whole, cracked or bleached flour	Malt (small amounts in cereal
Wheat germ	can usually be tolerated)
Farina	Graham flour
Gluten	Kasha
Rye	Dried peas or beans
Oats	Barley
Millet	Wheat Starch

Check with the company on any food product that contains the following words: flour, starch, emulsifiers, stabilizers or hydrolyzed vegetable protein. The product should not be used if the protein is wheat, rye, oats or barley. Companies are usually very cooperative about answering your questions, but be specific, as they offer only the information you request.

WHEAT

Bran	Malt
Bread crumbs	Cracker meal
Farina	Wheat germ

Flour; all-purpose, wheat, enriched graham, bread, cake, pastry, self-rising phosphates, wheat starch.

CORN

Corn oil—usually will not cause harm, but watch for any reaction while you use it. Don't discount the possibility that the problem can be the oil and not the food being prepared.

Corn sugar	Cornstarch
Cartose	Grits
Corn syrup	Hominy
Yeasts	Monosodium glutamate
Cerelose	Popcorn
Dyno	Caramel coloring
Sorbitol	Dextrose—very often means corn
Starch	

Most commercially canned fruits in syrup
White vinegar—it is distilled from corn
Most bacon and ham that is sugar-cured (some are not, check with company)
Baking powder (except Cellu cereal-free)
Powdered sugar (contains 3% cornstarch)
All commercially canned jelly, jam and preserves
All gum, mints, and candy
Many stickers, stamps, and envelopes use a corn substance for glue

Your doctor or health department can give you a very complete list of corn-containing products.

A more thorough list of corn-containing products is obtainable through your allergist or local Health Department.

MILK

Milk—whole, skimmed, dry, condensed, evaporated

Cream	Milk chocolate	Casein (the protein in milk)
Buttermilk	Nougat	Lactalbumin (curds and whey)
Cheese	Cottage cheese	
Custard	Junket	
Butter	Malted milk	

EGGS

Egg—yolk, white, whole or dried
Albumen (egg white)
Vitellin
Meringue
Ovamucin
Globulin

Eggnog
Ovovitellin
Mayonnaise
Ova mucoid
Livetin

CITRIC ACID

Any product with the word citric or citrate in the ingredient list on the label.
These foods contain citric acid:

Orange
Lemon
Citron
Kumquat
Lime

Grapefruit
Tangerine
Apricot, though not classified as a citrus
fruit is very high in citric acid content

CHEMICAL ADDITIVES

Food additives are becoming a greater problem for allergic Americans every day. It has been estimated that 12 per cent of Americans are allergic to them and it is becoming harder and harder to eliminate them from the diet. Antibiotics and chemicals given to animals, to fatten them, go into the meat. Chemical sprays on fruits and vegetables are very difficult to wash off completely. A list of the most volatile additives that require labeling on canned and otherwise-packaged goods follows:

Amaranth (Red Dye)
Tartrazine (Yellow Dye #5)
Salicylates (Aspirin Sensitivity—A
very thorough list is available
through doctors)
Sodium Nitrite
Sodium Benzoate
BHA
BHT
MSG (Monosodium Glutamate)
Iodine
Aniline (or Coal Tar Products)
Phenylethyl

FOOD SUBSTITUTES

FLOUR

When you become more sure of yourself in your new style of cooking you may wish to try developing your own recipes. All of the gluten-free flours may be interchanged, but the amounts that equal one cup of wheat flour vary greatly. This chart may help:

5/8 c. or 10 T. potato starch flour = 1 c. wheat flour

7/8 c. or 14 T. rice flour = 1 c. wheat flour

1 c. soybean flour and ¼ c. potato starch = 1 c. wheat flour (soybean flour *must* be used in combination with another flour)

When adding special flours to a recipe don't add all of the flour unless you have tried the recipe before. Very often the flour thickens fast. I've found that when you use no eggs it is best to thicken no more than to the consistency of a *normal* cake mix or your finished product will be very doughy.

For smaller amounts of flour use this substitution list:

½ T. potato starch flour = 1 T. wheat flour

½ T. rice flour = 1 T. wheat flour

½ T. arrowroot starch = 1 T. wheat flour

2   teasp. tapioca flour = 1 T. wheat flour

EGG

There are several ways that you can make up for a lack of eggs in the diet. Don't try to replace more than two eggs, or you won't have enough leavening activity.

1. Use Jolly Joan Egg Replacer – this has no egg derivatives.
2. Beat one minute extra for each egg missing. This incorporates more air to substitute for the leavening.
3. Add 1 extra teaspoon of baking power for each missing egg.
4. You can use 1 package of Knox gelatin as a binder.
5. In baked goods, use shortening instead of oil, because you can beat air into it better.
6. One mashed ripe banana can be used as a binder in place of one egg.

CITRIC ACID

Citric acid is used in many recipes to give a tangy flavor to the food. The food is more bland without it, but it can still be enjoyable. Use flavorings that you buy at the grocer's, and experiment. Do not use the citrus flavors because they usually contain oil from the plant.

MILK

Replacing milk in a recipe is quite simple. You can use water, juice or soybean milk. The texture and flavor is different with each. Water leaves the finished product with a coarser texture than formula. (Formula when used in this book refers to 1 can of soy base diluted with 1½ cans of water.) Remember not to boil puddings or sauces made with soybean milk because they will separate. You can, however, heat them until hot enough *almost* to boil without causing any harm to them. This temperature is sufficient to thicken a sauce, make gravy, or make a cream soup. You will have no difficulty baking cookies or cakes with soybean formula. In fact, it gives them a somewhat nutty flavor. The powdered soy milks (Fearn, Jolly Joan) don't have the pleasant flavor of the formula.

One other warning—rennet custards will not coagulate with any milk replacement. Tapioca flour is a good thickener for pudding.

CORN

Corn is a difficult food to eliminate completely from the diet because it is hidden in so many foods. Here are a few suggestions that may help:

1. Regular *baking powder* has cornstarch as an ingredient. It can be replaced in the following ways:
   a. By making your own baking powder.
      ¼ teaspoon baking soda
      ½ teaspoon cream of tartar
      This equals 1 teaspoon baking powder
   b. Using Cellu cereal-free baking powder in the normal amounts the recipe calls for.

2. *Powdered Sugar* contains 3% cornstarch but you can make your own from granulated sugar. Just pour sugar in your blender one cup at a time and blend until powdery. Don't keep your blender running the entire time it is blending because the motor heats up without liquid in the top. Blend a short time and allow to cool for about five minutes. Store any leftover sugar in a tightly covered container. This will cake much more easily than boxed powdered sugar, so sift or reblend it before using any that you have stored. This is a little bit grainier than store-bought powdered sugar. Several sizes of rice noodles and vermicelli are also available. (See list in back of book.)

3. There are a few brands of *brown sugar* that contain cornstarch, so be sure to read labels.

4. *Honey*—if sugar bothers your child, try *Tupelo Blossom Honey*, (available at health-food stores). This honey as a replacement is levulose, not glucose. Many children can tolerate any type of honey. I would suggest trying the less expensive honey found in the supermarket first. However, we found that Tupelo is the only kind David tolerates.

¾ c. honey = 1 c. sugar

Delete 3 T. liquid from recipe

Cookies made with honey retain their moisture and therefore store for a longer period of time.

ADDING VARIETY TO MENUS—Variety can be added to your menus by trying a few extra tricks:

1. Beat Rice Chex or Rice Krispies in the blender to make crumbs for breading meats or topping casseroles. These can be stored in a jar for future use.

2. If your child can tolerate gluten-free wheat starch, Cellu makes an excellent macaroni substitute, called Lo/Pro Pasta. It is very delicate, so be careful when you stir in the sauce.

3. A mixture called coconut-sesame seed meal, which is ground fine and has the flavor of nuts, is great in cookies or cakes even a toddler can enjoy.

4. Dip any cookie recipe in a cinnamon-sugar mixture before baking.

5. Cookies freeze well. Bake several kinds and freeze in mixed small packets so your child doesn't tire of one kind of cookie.

6. Make frosted cupcakes instead of a cake and freeze.

7. Bake bread and freeze before slicing. As needed, remove the bread from the freezer and slice what you want. Then return the unused portion to the freezer immediately.

8. Make small pancakes and use any leftovers as bread.

9. Breakfast can be less boring if you vary the flavor of his rice cereal. Try pouring on juice instead of formula, or use brown sugar instead of white. What about cinnamon sugar on top, or maple syrup?

I know that right now you are thinking that cooking with special flours, baking powder, egg replacers and such must be quite expensive. Not so! Usually you bake the cookies and bread only for the person on the diet. These flours go almost twice as far as wheat flour, as indicated in the substitution tables earlier in the chapter.

The only real expense is in the initial purchase, which can be kept at a minimum. I have found that the most important purchases are:

> Potato flour
> Rice flour
> Egg replacer
> Cereal-free baking powder
> Formula
> Knox gelatin
> Milk-free margarine
> Rice wafers
> For brand names see back of book.

If you buy these things, you can make most of the recipes in this book. Items except for formula should last about two months. Don't overstock because the flours especially are quite perishable and should be kept only for about three months. Keeping these suggestions in mind, you will find the expense minor when you begin to realize the results of your efforts.

Now, to get into some special areas and the recipes that will help you in feeding your allergic child!

7

Diarrhea Diet and Recipes

Most children with gastrointestinal allergy or malabsorption tend to get diarrhea very easily. We spent nine months controlling our son's diarrhea, but the results were worth the effort. Sure, we have setbacks occasionally but they aren't nearly as bad as they were in the beginning.

The most important effort you can make when your child has diarrhea is the forcing of fluids. If you can keep your child from dehydrating, you have won half the battle.

Signs of dehydration are:

1. Sunken eyes and protruding veins in face.
2. Hollowness of cheeks and temples and in infants depressed fontanelle (soft spot).
3. Dry, cherry-red lips.
4. Dry, thick coating on tongue.
5. Dryness of the skin. When you lightly pinch the skin the wrinkling remains raised, the skin's elasticity is gone.
6. Rise in temperature, along with poor fluid intake.
7. Scanty output of urine, with strong odor and dark color.
8. Listlessness—lies around an unusual amount.
9. Sudden weight loss.

If your child develops any of these symptoms in connection with diarrhea, be sure to notify your doctor and continue forcing fluids.

Our baby had vomiting (not spitting up—vomiting is more profuse, makes the baby cry afterwards, and doesn't stop after one or two times) along with diarrhea, and there were times when the doctor would say, "Don't give him anything but water for twenty-four hours. Then report to me by phone." Sometimes the doctor may order electrolytes added to fluid to replace those lost by vomiting and diarrhea. It is very important, for your own peace of mind, to have a pediatrician in whom you have great faith and who knows your child well. If your pediatrician has several partners, ask for the same doctor as much as possible so your child will be well known to him, and observations can be better evaluated. It is very difficult for a doctor to determine the severity of an illness when he has not seen the child well and therefore has no basis for comparison. It is very hard for a parent to take all food away from a baby and give him nothing but water. Faith in your doctor is the only way you can accept such an order. We were afraid and sure the baby would die without food; but once we were confident that the doctor knew what he was doing it was easier to follow his instructions.

Usually, within a few hours, the vomiting stopped and the baby would begin taking water well. He went through this water diet several times and has suffered no ill effect. Let me caution you, however, if the vomiting doesn't stop within a few hours be sure to call your doctor before the twenty-four hours are up because sometimes vomiting is irreversible without medication and constant vomiting can hasten dehydration.

Before you panic, however, there are several home remedies you can try before calling the doctor. In all cases of vomiting it is best to wait one hour after the last upchucking before you give ANYTHING by mouth. AND ANYTHING INCLUDES EVEN A SIP OF WATER! Once the stomach begins to reject food, there is an almost mechanical cycle started, and until the stomach is permitted to quiet, chances are excellent that no matter what you put in it is going to come right back out. So allow the stomach to rest for at least an hour and then try one of the following:

1. Weak tea, slightly sweetened, but no milk. Give one teaspoon every five minutes for half an hour, then small sips every five minutes for the next hour or so.
2. Warm or room-temperature club soda with a small amount of sugar added to flavor it. This is given in the same manner as the tea above.
3. Apple pop (See recipe on page 78.)

There are two other very good remedies, but they may cause problems with some children's diets. Do not use them if your child is allergic to any of the ingredients.

1. Coca-cola syrup (available from your druggist) does contain corn. Give one teaspoon every fifteen minutes for an hour, then sips of tea, club soda, apple pop or water. Lollipops are also good at this time.
2. Warm or room-temperature ginger ale—contains both citric acid and corn, but if these are tolerated by your child, ginger ale is very good used in the same manner as the weak tea.

Avoid putting large quantities of anything, liquid or solid, into an already queasy stomach, and keep the child on a light diet for the rest of the day after vomiting is brought under control. Once the vomiting is controlled, you can turn your attention to controlling the diarrhea.

Our doctor gave us the diarrhea diet slip that he uses for all his patients and I adapted it to my needs. This is the diet that worked for David.

Diluted half-strength formula	Cellu or Holgrain rice wafers
Apple juice popsicles	Raw scraped apple (not applesauce)

*Apple and coconut sauce   Potato, baked
*Gelatin dessert   *Rice water
Apple juice   *Cinnamon tea
Rice   *Apple pop
Rice cereal   Bananas
Lean meat   *Beef tea
                                  The recipes for (*) foods follow:

APPLE AND COCONUT SAUCE

Prepare in blender:
    6   raw apples, quartered
    ¼ c. shredded coconut
    Heinz Rice Cereal to thicken (about ¼ c.)
    ½ c. water
1. Put water in blender and start.
2. Add apples one by one until chopped.
3. Add coconut.
4. Add rice cereal to thicken.

Makes six ½-cup servings.
** P. 0.1 C.1.3 F. 1 Cal. 74.6

GELATIN DESSERT

    1   T. unflavored gelatin
    ½ c. cold water
    ⅓ c. sugar
    ⅛ t. salt
    1   c. boiling water
1. Sprinkle gelatin on cold water to soften.
2. Add remaining ingredients and stir until thoroughly dissolved.
3. Add variation below and chill. (I use 3 oz. disposable plastic cups or covered jar to take with me.)

Makes 4 to 6 servings.
P. 1.1 C. 15.0 F.− Cal. 67

Variations: Add−
    ½ c. cooked rice
    ½ raw chopped apples

(Including gel) P. 1.6 C. 252.0 F. trace Cal. 110.0

**The number values for P. (Protein) C. (Carbohydrate) and F. (Fat) are always figures in *grams*. A − after one of these letters indicates that there is none of that substance in the recipe. Unless otherwise noted these number values refer to one portion servings.

SLUSH

½ c. allowable juice
5   ice cubes

1. Place juice in blender and start.
2. Drop in ice cubes one at a time until all are crushed. The new slush mugs that you freeze and then add juice to also work well.

Computed using apple juice – P. trace C. 17.0 F.– Cal. 63.0

JUICE POPSICLES

2 cups juice poured into cups or popsicle molds and freeze or, to make less drippy popsicles add:

1   T. unflavored gelatin
½ c. juice to soften gel
¼ c. sugar
1   c. boiling water—stir until mixture dissolves
1   c. juice

Pour into molds and freeze. Store leftover mixture in refrigerator. Serve as gel.

Makes about 12 molds.

Computed using apple juice – P. 0.4 C. 4.7 F.– Cal. 20.0

BEEF TEA

1   lb. chopped or ground beef—fresh, for mold allergy
2   c. cold water
½ t. salt

1. Place meat in a jar and add water.
2. Allow to stand for 1 hour.
3. Place jar in a saucepan of cold water with a cloth on the bottom of the pan under the glass to keep the jar from breaking.
4. Heat over low heat, being careful not to let boil. Keep below boiling for 2 hours.
5. Slowly increase heat sufficiently to turn the beef tea to a deep chocolate color.
6. Strain and add salt.

Never allow to boil either in making or reheating.

Makes 2 servings.

P. 52.5 C. trace F. 42.5 Cal. 612.0

RICE WATER
(for diarrhea)

2   quarts water
½ c. regular rice
1. Boil water and add rice. Boil ½ hour.
2. Strain and reserve water.
3. Cool.
4. Pour in bottles, adding ½ t. sugar per 8 ounces.
This is very good for a baby and works very well.

(Accurate only if rice is eaten also)
P. 2.0 C. 22.0 F.– Cal. 102.5

CINNAMON TEA
(for diarrhea)

2   sticks cinnamon
2   quarts water
Sugar to sweeten
1. Boil mixture for about 45 minutes.
2. Add sugar to sweeten.
3. Cool down for a child.
This is an old remedy for diarrhea but it works well. Can even be used by adults and served hot.

BANANA MILK
(for diarrhea)

Add 1 T. Nanana Banana Flakes to an 8 oz. bottle of dilute formula; this will hasten the development of formed stools.

APPLE POP

Add ¾ c. apple juice and ¼ club soda and stir with a swizzle stick.
Use as you normally would use ginger ale.

P. – C. 25.5 F.– Cal. 93.6

FRUIT OR VEGETABLE JUICE WITH GELATIN

1   T. unflavored gelatin
¾ c. cold juice to soften gel (apple juice)
¾ c. chilled juice
1. Soften gel in top of a small double boiler.
2. Stir over boiling water until thoroughly dissolved.
3. Remove from heat and add chilled juice and ice, if desired, for cold drink.

(Total for recipe) P. 6 C. 51.0 F. trace Cal. 212.5

8

Baby and Toddler Diet and Recipes

According to our pediatric allergist, a baby digests food differently from an adult. Adults assimilate only the amino acid (the usable part of the food after it is digested) from their intestines, which causes a less severe reaction to the food to which they are allergic. A baby, however, assimilates the entire food into his blood stream because the normal holes in the intestines through which the food is absorbed are larger than in adults. This total absorption causes the allergy-prone child to have a greater exposure to the allergen (the part of the food that causes his allergy problem).

Your child will never have a reaction to a food the first time he eats it because he has no antibodies formed to it until he has eaten the food at least once. Antibodies prevent the child from having a reaction to a particular food; but they are formed by exposing the body to the food in very small amounts at a time. The second time he eats it, however, he may have a reaction. To prevent early allergy to a food, keep your baby's diet simple during the first two years. Babies can live happily with a very limited diet, so don't expose them to unnecessary allergies.

It is often quite difficult to find prepared baby foods that an allergic baby can eat. In this event, the most important appliance in your kitchen is a blender. These suggestions might help you to prepare your own baby food.

MEAT—Meat is usually not a problem to the baby unless he is allergic to a particular meat or can't tolerate fat. The broth is a little fatty in some brands of baby food, so try several different brands to see which is best tolerated by your baby. If you find that you can't use any of the prepared meats try this:

BABY MEAT
Blend ½ cup of water with about 1 cup, boiled until tender, meat that has been trimmed of all fat and gristle. Blend until fine-textured. If it seems too thick, add extra water; if too thin, add extra meat or rice cereal until the desired consistency is reached.

VEGETABLES—Use prepared vegetables with nothing but water and salt added. Read canned vegetable labels carefully since some have milk or MSG added.

FRUITS—This is where you will run into the most problems with citric acid. Many prepared baby fruits have orange juice or citric acid added. You can buy, in the dietetic department of some supermarkets or health-food stores, water or juice packed (Cellu, Natur Made) fruit in cans. Make sure it is not artificially sweetened. Read the label carefully because some of the juices are from a different fruit than is in the can. These fruits can be blended in a blender with about ¼ cup of the drained liquid.

If you have more food than you can use, freeze the leftovers in ice cube trays; when frozen, remove and pack in plastic bags. Later, one or two cubes can be thawed with heated water. In this way, you can add variety to your child's diet without wasting any of the food.

JUICES—Read labels carefully. Many baby juices have orange juice or citric acid added. You may want to dilute juices by half because they are sometimes too concentrated and cause the child to cough or choke. An older baby can often drink regular canned juice but there are very few juices that *do not* contain citric acid. You might try making homemade juice from fresh fruit.

HOMEMADE JUICE
1. Wash, core or stem and crush fruit and place in a cheesecloth sack.
2. Add 1 cup of water for every 4 cups of prepared fruit in the sack and place in a large pan.
3. Set the bag of fruit in the pan of water and simmer for 15 minutes.
4. Remove the cheesecloth bag to a colander and allow it to drain into the cooking pan for about an hour without squeezing.
5. Pour the juice into a covered jar and let it stand in the refrigerator for 24 hours, then re-strain it.
6. Keep refrigerated, or freeze into cubes to use as desired.

There are several recipes that my toddler enjoyed even though he was on a very restricted diet. These children enjoy finger foods just as much as other toddlers do although they can't have pretzels, rusk, and arrowroot cookies. These recipes may be of interest to you.

BREAKFAST
You may find that your child is becoming tired of the same old rice cereal taste that he gets every morning. This may be a real treat for him.

LUMBERJACK'S BREAKFAST

1 c. Rice Chex
1 c. Puffed Rice
1 c. Rice Krispies
½ c. shredded coconut
½ c. sesame seeds
¾ c. maple syrup
¼ c. brown sugar
1 c. shortening or oil

1. Combine dry ingredients, except sugar, in a bowl.
2. Bring syrup, sugar, and shortening to a rolling boil in a saucepan.
3. Pour the syrup mixture over the cereal and coat well, stirring carefully.
4. Spread the cereal on two cookie sheets and bake at 300 degrees for about 20-30 minutes until browned and dry.
5. Break apart when cooled and reserve some large pieces for him to eat in his hand.
6. Store the remainder in a plastic bag or tightly covered container when completely cooled.
7. Serve with a milk substitute.

Makes 24 ½-cup servings.
P. 10.4 C. 11.9 F. 0.4 Cal. 140.4

CINNAMON CHEX

¼ c. milk-free margarine
1 t. cinnamon
3 T. sugar
1 c. Rice Chex

1. Melt margarine, add cinnamon and sugar and mix well.
2. Add Rice Chex and coat thoroughly, stirring gently.
3. Serve immediately.

Serves 3.
P. 0.6 C. 18.9 F. 15.3 Cal. 214.3

RICE FLOUR PANCAKES

1 c. rice flour
1½ t. cereal-free baking powder
3 T. sugar or 1 T. Tupelo Blossom honey to facilitate browning

    ½ t. salt
1   t. egg replacer
2   T. water
1   c. prepared soy base (dilution used in this book is always 1 can
     soy base to 1½ cans water)
3   T. melted milk-free margarine
1. Heat lightly greased griddle.
2. Stir together the dry ingredients in a medium sized bowl.
3. Combine liquid ingredients and add to the dry ingredients.
4. Mix well.
5. Drop batter by heaping tablespoons onto the griddle. Cook on one side
   until full of bubbles. Turn and brown the other side.
Very tasty if you cook them small and refrigerate any leftovers to use as bread.

                                              Makes 12 four-inch pancakes.
                                          P. 1.4 C. 16.7 F. 3.6 Cal. 96.6

RICE MIX WAFFLES

1   c. Jolly Joan rice mix (available in health food stores)
1   t. egg replacer
2   T. water
1   c. formula or water
1   T. oil
1. Combine all ingredients.
2. Stir until batter is smooth.
3. When waffle iron starts to smoke, pour in batter.
4. Waffle is done when steaming from waffle iron stops.
Freeze leftover cooked waffles and reheat in the toaster as needed.

                                              Makes 4 small waffles.
                                          P. 2.8 C. 34.3 F. 5.7 Cal. 199.6

SYRUP

Use pure maple syrup, cinnamon sugar, or the following recipe:
    1   c. brown sugar
    ¼ c. water
    ½ t. cinnamon
    ½ t. vanilla
1. Mix together in saucepan.
2. Boil five minutes and serve warm.
                                    (Total) P. — C. 208 F. — Cal. 800

    Most commercial syrups contain corn syrup or caramel coloring. However,
you can use pure maple syrup, honey, or *Coconut Island* free-flowing Coconut
Syrup (Agar). *Yinnies* Rice Syrup (malted barley).

FRUITS

FRUIT GELATIN DESSERT

1 Bar of Agar Agar (a gum)
3 c. Allowable Juice
1. Soak Agar Agar in cold juice, in a saucepan until soft.
2. Bring to a low boil for 15 minutes.
3. Remove from heat and cool slightly.
4. Add desired variations.
5. Chill until firm in molds, cups or jars.

VARIATIONS
Add 1 cup of chopped fruit.
Add 1 4¾ oz. jar of baby food fruit.
Add shredded, sliced or chopped raw or cooked vegetables for a beautiful salad.

Serves 6.

APRICOT SHAKE

¼ c. undiluted soy base
¼ c. cold water
1-3 oz. jar strained apricots
4 ice cubes
1. Combine all ingredients except the ice in a blender.
2. Start blender and drop in ice cubes one at a time until all ice is crushed.
3. Serve at once.

Makes 1½ cups.
P. 2.1 C. 22.7 F. 4.2 Cal. 137.6

APPLESAUCE

2 tart apples, washed, cored and sliced
Water to cover
Sugar to taste
½ t. cinnamon (optional)
1. Place apples and water in a small saucepan.
2. Cover and cook over low heat until soft, 8-10 minutes.
3. Sweeten and stir until sugar is dissolved.
4. Serve hot or cold.

Serves 2.
P. 1 C. 61 F. − Cal. 230.0

STEWED APPLES

    4   medium cooking apples
       ½ c. sugar
    2   c. boiling water
    Dash of nutmeg or cinnamon

1. Wash apples and cut into eighths, peel and core.
2. Place in cold water.
3. Combine sugar and boiling water in a shallow saucepan and stir over low heat until sugar is dissolved.
4. Add cinnamon or nutmeg, if desired.
5. Drain apples and cook in the syrup mixture until transparent.
6. Add boiling water to syrup if it thickens too much during cooking.

Serves 4.
P. – C. 42.9 F. – Cal. 166.2

STEWED PEARS

    4   medium pears
    4 -8 cloves, as desired
       ½ c. boiling water
       ½ c. sugar

1. Wash and peel pears, remove core if desired.
2. Stud each pear with cloves and arrange in a 10″ covered frypan.
3. Sprinkle with sugar and add water.
4. Cover and cook over very low heat until tender when poked with a toothpick. Serve hot or cold.

Serves 4.
P. 1.0 C. 89.0 F. 1.0 Cal. 200.0

STEWED RHUBARB

    2   pounds rhubarb
    1   c. sugar

1. Trim rhubarb removing leaves and stem ends of stalks.
2. Wash and cut into 1-inch pieces.
3. Place in top of double boiler.
4. Add sugar and cook, covered, over boiling water until rhubarb is soft.

Serves 6.
P. 1.0 C. 98.0 F. trace Cal. 385.0

FRUIT PUDDING

    2   c. fruit juice
    2   T. Cellu tapioca starch flour
       ¼ c. sugar
    1   c. quick-cooking rice

1. Pour 1½ cups juice in a saucepan.
2. Mix tapioca flour with remainder of the juice and add to saucepan.
3. Add sugar and mix well.
4. Heat over medium heat, stirring constantly. When liquid becomes clear and boils slightly, remove from heat.
5. Add rice and cover for 5 minutes.
6. Pour into individual dishes.

Serves 6.
P. 0.7 C. 26.7 F. – Cal. 51.1

LUNCH

Everyone enjoys a good lunch, including your toddler. Here are a few suggestions that you may find helpful for a change of pace.

GRILLED PEANUT BUTTER SANDWICH (contains legumes)

2   slices Rice Bread*
Milk-free margarine
Old-fashioned peanut butter (homogenized contains corn)
1. Spread peanut butter in center of bread.
2. Spread margarine on outside, both sides.
3. Grill (as grilled cheese) at about 350 degrees to melt the peanut butter.

Serves 1.
P. 9.0 C. 62.0 F. 18.2 Cal. 439.8

Makes a tasty lunch with a soup that is allowed.

CELERY SOUP

½ c. diced celery
2   slices onion
½ t. salt
½ c. water
½ c. undiluted soy base
Dash of pepper
1   T. minced parsley
1. Combine all but soy base and parsley and cook over low heat until celery is tender, about 5 minutes.
2. Add soy base to above mixture and heat almost to boiling. DO NOT BOIL.
3. Serve garnished with parsley.

Serves 1.
P. 5.2 C. 25.1 F. 4.4 Cal. 160.8

*See index for page numbers

BLENDER PEA SOUP (contains legumes)

1   pkg. frozen peas (12 oz.)—break apart and set aside to thaw.
Place following ingredients in the blender in the order given.
   1   c. prepared soy base
   1   T. rice flour
   2   T. milk-free margarine
    ½ t. salt
    ½ t. nutmeg
    ⅛ t. pepper
   1   small onion, quartered

1. ALWAYS COVER BLENDER BEFORE STARTING AND STOPPING MOTOR TO AVOID SPLASHING.
2. After adding the above in order, cover blender and turn on.
3. Continue to blend while gradually adding half of the peas. Use rubber spatula to scrape down sides so ingredients are evenly blended. Blend about 1½ minutes and empty mixture into saucepan.
4. Pour 1 more cup of prepared formula into the blender and gradually add the remaining peas. Blend 1 minute.
5. Stir into mixture that is already in the saucepan and heat very hot (DO NOT BOIL). Stir occasionally. You can add sliced franks, Vienna sausages or diced ham (mold).

Makes five ¾ c. servings.
P. 4.8 C. 14.4 F. 6.4 Cal. 134.8

POTATO SOUP

   1   medium potato, diced
   2   T. minced onion
    ¼ t. salt
    ¾ c. prepared soy base
   1   T. milk-free margarine
   1   T. minced parsley
   Dash of pepper

1. Put potato and water to cover in a small saucepan.
2. Add onion and salt.
3. Cover and cook until potato is tender.
4. Place in blender and add margarine and formula.
5. Blend until smooth.
6. Reheat and serve garnished with parsley.

Serves 1.
P. 5.6 C. 30.5 F. 17.8 Cal. 300.4

TODDLER MEAT COOKIES

2   T. shortening
¾ t. salt
¾ t. baking soda
1 ½ t. cream of tartar
2   T. sugar
1   3-oz. jar of strained or junior meat (not ham—too greasy)
2   c. Heinz rice cereal

1. Combine all ingredients except cereal and stir until well mixed and fluffy.
2. Add cereal all at once and work into the above until well mixed. (Dough will be gummy.)
3. Drop from spoon and pat down.
4. Bake at 450 degrees for 10-12 minutes.

Very good, not messy, good as a first finger food.

Makes about 14 cookies.
P. 1.4 C. 5.9 F. 2.5 Cal. 52.0

CHICKEN VEGETABLE WITH RICE SOUP

1   3-pound chicken, cut up
4   c. water
1 ½ t. salt
1   small onion
Celery leaves
1   parsnip
1   carrot
¼ t. marjoram
1   t. parsley flakes
¾ c. raw rice

1. Boil chicken, water, salt, marjoram and celery leaves in covered pan for 1 hour.
2. Remove chicken. Skin and bone it and cut up in pieces.
3. Strain liquid and replace in pan with chicken.
4. Add remaining ingredients and simmer until tender.
5. Salt to taste.

Serves 6.
(1 c. serving) P. 16.4 C. 18.1 F. 1.3 Cal. 152.8

RICE WAFERS

¼ c. milk-free margarine (soft-spread—stick type too salty)
¼ c. sugar
1   t. egg replacer
2   T. water
¾ c. sifted rice flour

1. Cream margarine and sugar.
2. Add egg replacer and stir in flour.
3. Roll out between two sheets of plastic wrap, as thin as possible. Cut with knife or cookie cutters.

4. Bake on nonstick cookie sheet 400 degrees for about 8 minutes, until golden brown.

These would be good with soup for lunch.

Makes 30 wafers.

P. 0.3 C. 4.8 F. 1.5 Cal. 33.2

DESSERTS

SPICE STICKS

1   c. rice flour
½ t. salt
⅓ c. shortening
2   T. sugar
1   t. cinnamon
Cold water

1. Sift flour and salt together and cut in shortening until mixture resembles coarse meal.
2. Add cold water a few drops at a time, until dough is just moist enough to hold together. Chill overnight.
3. Roll into a rectangle and sprinkle with mixture of cinnamon and sugar.
4. Fold ends of dough into center, then fold through center to make 4 layers.
5. Roll out again to ¼-inch thickness.
6. Fold again as before.
7. Roll out again to 1/8-inch thickness.
8. Cut into narrow sticks and bake in a very hot oven (450 degrees) for 8 to 10 minutes.

These could be cut into animal shapes.

Makes 4-5 doz. 4" sticks.

P. 0.2 C. 2.4 F. 1.2 Cal. 21.5

FRUIT COOKIES

¼ c. shortening
¼ c. sugar
¼ t. salt
1 ½ t. cereal-free baking powder
2   c. Heinz rice cereal
1   4 ¾-oz. jar strained baby fruit

1. Cream shortening and sugar thoroughly.
2. Mix all ingredients, except cereal, and beat until fluffy.
3. Add all of cereal at once and mix well.
4. Form dough into small balls and place on a lightly greased cookie sheet and press very thin with a fork.

5. Bake at 350 degrees for 10-12 minutes or until light brown.
6. Remove to a rack and cool well. Store in a closed container.

Makes 20 cookies.
P. 0.3 C. 6.6 F. 3.0 Cal. 53.7

APPLESAUCE COOKIES

   ½ c. shortening
1   c. sugar or ¾ c. Tupelo honey (inerease flour slightly)
   ½ c. applesauce
3   c. rice flour
1 ½ t. cereal-free baking powder
   ¼ t. vanilla
   ¼ t. cinnamon (optional)

1. Cream sugar and shortening thoroughly.
2. Stir in applesauce and blend well.
3. Blend in all dry ingredients.
4. Drop by teaspoonfuls onto a lightly greased baking sheet.
5. Bake at 375 degrees for 10-12 minutes.

Makes about 4½ dozen.
P. 0.7 C. 11.1 F. 2.1 Cal. 56

FRUITY RICE PUDDING

⅔ c. uncooked quick-cooking rice
1 ¼ c. water
   ¼ t. salt
1   junior-size jar of strained fruit
2 ½ T. brown sugar
1   T. milk-free margarine

1. Combine all ingredients in a saucepan and simmer, covered, for seven minutes.
2. Fluff gently with a fork twice during cooking.
3. Remove from heat and let stand, covered, five minutes.
4. Serve warm.

Serves 4.
P. 0.7 C. 27.8 F. 0.5 Cal. 121.1

PEAR GELATIN

1   T. unflavored gelatin, softened in ¼ c. cold water
   ¾ c. hot water
   ¼ c. cold water
   ½ c. pear juice

⅛ t. ginger
½ t. salt
2 c. cut-up canned pears

1. Add hot water to softened gelatin, stir until dissolved.
2. Add cold water, juice, ginger, salt and stir well.
3. Add pears when gelatin is partially set.
4. Refrigerate until firm.

Serves 4.
P. 2.0 C. 23.5 F. trace Cal. 94.5

BAKED CINNAMON APPLES

4 apples, peeled halfway down, washed and cored
1 ½ c. sugar
¾ c. water
2 two-inch sticks of cinnamon

1. Place apples in a deep baking dish.
2. Combine sugar and water and pour over apples.
3. Drop cinnamon sticks into baking dish.
4. Bake at 350 degrees for about 50 minutes, basting often with syrup in dish. Apples are done when they are tender when pierced with a fork, yet firm enough to hold their shape.

Serves 4.
P. trace C. 90.0 F. trace Cal. 370.0

POPPED APPLE

4 apples, cored and peeled one-half inch down from stem.
2 c. club soda
¼ c. sugar
4 T. unsweetened black cherry concentrate (Vita-Nutri or Nu-Life black cherry concentrate)

1. Mix soda, sugar and black cherry concentrate gently so as not to lose all of the carbonation.
2. Fill individual custard cups half full of the mixture.
3. Place apple in cup, turning top (peeled) side down.
4. Pour remaining liquid over apples to nearly fill cups.
5. Bake at 350 degrees for 45 minutes.

Serves 4.
P. trace C. 31.0 F. trace Cal. 120.0

HOME-FRIED APPLES

2 T. milk-free margarine
6 medium apples, cored and sliced
3 T. sugar
½ t. cinnamon

1. Melt margarine in a skillet.
2. Add apples, sugar and cinnamon and cook over medium heat for about 15 minutes until done.
3. Turn over during cooking.

Makes 4-6 servings.
P. trace C. 36.0 F. 2.0 Cal. 162.5

VANILLA PUDDING

2   T. tapioca starch
¼ c. sugar
⅛ t. salt
¾ c. undiluted soy base
¾ c. water
½ t. vanilla

1. Combine tapioca starch, sugar and salt in top of double boiler.
2. Gradually add soy base and water, stirring well.
3. Cook over boiling water, stirring constantly, until thickened and smooth— about 5 minutes.
4. Cover and cook for 15 minutes, stirring occasionally.
5. Remove from heat, stir in vanilla.
6. Pour into serving dishes and chill.

Serves 3.
P. 4.1 C. 56.9 F. 8.5 Cal. 317.5

BUTTERSCOTCH PUDDING

1   c. soy base, undiluted
1   c. hot water
¾ c. brown sugar
3   T. tapioca starch
½ t. salt
1   T. vanilla

1. Combine tapioca starch, sugar and salt in the top of a double boiler.
2. Add formula and water, mix until all lumps are gone.
3. Cook over boiling water, stirring constantly.
4. Cook until thickened, about 5 minutes.
5. Cover and cook for another 10-15 minutes, stirring occasionally until thick.
6. Add vanilla and pour into serving dishes.
7. Refrigerate and serve.

Serves 3.
P. 5.8 C. 81.1 F. 11.3 Cal. 444.2

APRICOT PUDDING

1   pound can of apricots, pitted
⅔ c. quick-cooking rice, uncooked
¼ t. salt
Cinnamon

1 T. shortening
1 t. vanilla

1. Pit and quarter apricots.
2. In a one-quart casserole, combine rice, salt, vanilla, apricots and juice.
3. Sprinkle wtih cinnamon and dot with shortening.
4. Bake at 350 degrees for 20-25 minutes. Serve warm.

If you refrigerate cooked rice pudding, the rice hardens.

Serves 4.
P. 0.9 C. 20.2 F. 3.0 Cal. 114.1

APPLE TARTS

Crust

½ c. Cellu grainless mix
1 T. shortening
1 ½ T. warm water

1. Combine ingredients in a mixing bowl.
2. Work for a short time in your hands to form a smooth ball.
3. Roll out between plastic wrap and cut into 16 1½-inch squares.

Filling

½ c. applesauce
¼ t cinnamon
½ t sugar

1. Combine ingredients and mix well.
2. Place the mixture on half of squares of pie dough. Cover with the remaining squares.
3. Seal edges with fingers, prick tops and sprinkle with sugar.
4. Bake at 325 degrees for about 15 minutes.

Very nice for lunchbox dessert, but very moist, crumbles easily.

Makes about 8 tarts.
P. 1.1 C. 6.6 F. 2.8 Cal. 56.0

SPREADS

PEAR BUTTER

2 c. firm ripe pears; peeled, cored and cut in small pieces.
1 c. sugar
⅛ t. ginger
¼ t. cinnamon

1. Combine all ingredients and simmer for two hours, stirring frequently to prevent scorching, until mixture is quite thick. Serve as jam. Makes about 1 cup.

(Total) P. 1.0 C. 242.0 F. 1.0 Cal. 1000.0

HONEY BUTTER

2   T. honey
½ c. milk-free margarine
1. Combine ingredients in a small bowl.
2. Beat with mixer until fluffy. Makes about 2/3 cup.
Very tasty on rice wafers, rice crackers or pancakes.

(Total) P. trace C. 17.0 F. 110.4 Cal. 444.0

PEANUT BUTTER SUBSTITUTES

HAIN makes three:
Sesame Seed Butter
Sunflower Seed Butter
Sesame Tahini

TAHINI HONEY

½ c. Sesame Tahini
½ c. Honey
1. Combine and mix well.
2. Store in a jar to use as a sandwich spread.

FRUIT JAM (AGAR AGAR)

2 bars of Agar Agar
3 c. fruit juice
2 jars of strained baby fruit or ½ c. chopped canned fruit, drained
1. Soak Agar Agar in juice until soft.
2. Bring to a boil.
3. Slow boil for 10 minutes, add fruit and boil 5 minutes more, stirring to mix fruit thoroughly.
4. Pour into a jar and refrigerate.

9

Special Diet Food the Entire Family Will Enjoy

Believe it or not, it really isn't difficult to cook for the entire family with this diet. Just don't tell anyone what is in the sauces, casseroles, gravy or soup. Actually, the diet is quite high in protein and vitamins. The flavors are quite good in many of the main-dish recipes also. Soybean formula in place of milk lends a nutty flavor to a casserole or soup. You can get real raves for your gravy when you use rice flour or potato starch. Rice flour especially brings out a meatier flavor than wheat flour and isn't lumpy, so you're an expert on the first try!

If your child's diet is restricted in the use of vegetables, experiment with those he can have. You will be surprised at some of the flavors. When you make soup, have you ever considered using celery leaves, lettuce, parsnips, green pepper, or beets? Meat dipped in soybean formula and breaded with potato flour takes on a crispy and delicious flavor when oven-fried. Experiment with spices to vary your meals in flavor. Plain baked or boiled potatoes with broiled meat is the "ideal" for a special diet.

Here are some suggestions for spices and the foods they complement.

BEEF AND VEAL—allspice, basil, celery seed, cinnamon, curry, fennel, dill, garlic, marjoram, onion.

LAMB—dill, allspice, basil, cinnamon, cumin, curry, fennel, garlic, ginger, oregano, parsley, peppermint, rosemary, sage, savory, tarragon, thyme.

PORK—allspice, basil, celery seed, cinnamon, cumin curry, dill, garlic, ginger, marjoram, paprika, rosemary, sage, tarragon, thyme.

FISH AND POULTRY—basil, bay, celery seed, curry, garlic, ginger, onion, oregano, paprika, parsley, rosemary, sage, sesame seed, savory, tarragon.

POTATO DISHES—bay, caraway, celery seeds, chervil, chives, paprika, poppy seed, rosemary, tarragon, onion.

SOUPS—bay leaf, basil, garlic powder, onion, parsley, sage, thyme.

Cooking for someone on a restricted diet helps you cook with more imagination. You are forced to try new foods that you may never have come into contact with before. I have been surprised at how the rest of my family has responded to many of the diet recipes. I have had requests from my husband and children for a particular food. In fact, some of the recipes have been prepared for company and accepted very well. I've even been asked for the recipes! Be sure to write down any recipe that your family enjoys, including any changes you may have made. If you create a recipe, be sure to write it down right away otherwise it may be lost forever. If you are like me, you forget very easily what you did to the food that was different. Sometimes a minor change is all that is required to make a recipe more enjoyable. Remember the recipes in this book are only ideas to get you started. Look up your family favorites and see if they can be adapted using the information on substitutions furnished in chapter 6.

MEATS
Cook all roasts in cooking bags. They save the juices and help cook flavor into the meat. Follow the directions given on the package.

LEG OF LAMB
(Buy whole leg of lamb and have it cut in half. It is less expensive this way. Freeze one half for future use). Cook as follows:

1. Place unseasoned lamb into a cooking bag. You can add seasoning if you prefer. See list on previous page.

2. Bake at 300 degrees for about 2-3 hours until the meat begins to leave the bone.

3. Break bag to release juices and make gravy.*

Very good served with mint jelly. Very juicy and moist, and makes very good gravy.

Use leftovers for shepherd's pie.*

If you prefer to cook lamb in an open pan, coffee with seasonings added makes an excellent baste.

(3 oz. slice) P. 20.0 C. — F. 20.0 Cal. 265.0

Since bouillon cubes and canned bouillon or consomme contain ingredients not allowed on many allergy diets, here is a very useful recipe for bouillon that also provides your evening meal.

BOILED DINNER

1   4-pound rump roast
4   pounds soup bones
1   veal knuckle—cracked
4 ½ qts. water

*See index for page numbers.

1   large whole onion with 2 cloves inserted
1   bay leaf
 ¼ t. thyme
2   T. salt
2   stalks celery
1   turnip
4   carrots
1. Clean vegetables and cut up as desired.
2. Place meat, bones, salt, in a large soup kettle.
3. Add water and bring to a boil over high heat.
4. Lower heat and simmer for two hours, skimming the foam off frequently.
5. Add spices and vegetables, and continue simmering for an additional 1½ hours. Skim fat from top.
6. Serve meat and vegetables as main course.
7. Refrigerate broth and skim solidified fat from the surface.
8. Strain and freeze broth to use as soup base or bouillon as desired. Any leftover meat scraps can also be cut up and frozen for future use in soups.

Serves 5.
P. 98.9 C. 7.7 F. 68.5 Cal. 1064.1

BRAISED VEAL SHOULDER

3-5 pounds of boned and rolled veal shoulder
    salt, pepper and rice flour
1   T. shortening
1. Rub meat with the salt, pepper and flour mixture.
2. Brown on all sides in hot shortening.
3. Place meat on a rack in a deep pan and cover.
4. Roast in oven at 350 degrees for about 3 hours.
5. Make gravy with drippings.

Makes 16 3-oz. servings.
P. 18.0 C. trace F. 14.0 Cal. 205.0

BAKED SHOULDER OF LAMB

1   boned and rolled lamb shoulder roast
2   T. shortening
1   t. salt
 ¼ t. pepper
1   c. water
8   potatoes, peeled and sliced
1   small onion, thinly sliced
2   T. milk-free margarine
1   T. chopped parsley
1. Grease large baking dish and heavy skillet.
2. Put meat in skillet and cook until meat is browned on all sides.
3. Season with salt and pepper and place meat in baking dish.

4. Add water to skillet and bring to a boil.
5. Surround meat with potatoes and onion and pour liquid from skillet over potatoes and onion.
6. Dot with margarine.
7. Bake at 400 degrees for 1 hour, basting occasionally.
8. Cut meat into thin slices and arrange slices in center of baking dish. Sprinkle with parsley. Serve hot.

Serves 4.
P. 10.5 C. 46.5 F. 10.2 Cal. 310.2

CHICKEN CROQUETTES

1 T. oil
2 T. tapioca starch
½ c. chicken broth
¾ c. cooked chicken, ground
½ t. salt
1 c. Rice Chex or Rice Krispies, crushed

1. Combine oil, tapioca and broth. Cook over medium heat to make sauce.
2. Add the other ingredients. If mixture is too liquid add some of the crushed cereal.
3. Cool the above mixture in refrigerator until firm enough to mold.
4. Shape into croquettes.
5. Dip in remaining cereal and bake at 400 degrees about 30 minutes

Serves 4.
P. 10.9 C. 9.3 F. 5.0 Cal. 131.6

LAMB PATTIES

2 pounds ground lamb
Salt
Parsley flakes

1. Shape lamb into patties.
2. Salt and sprinkle with parsley.
3. Broil for 20 minutes, turning once.

Serves 6
P. 16.6 C. — F. 10.6 Cal. 266.6

OVEN-FRIED CHICKEN

1 frying chicken, cut up
½ c. potato flour
¼ t. nutmeg
1 t. salt
½ t sweet basil
¼ c. undiluted milk substitute
Dots of milk-free margarine

1. Mix dry ingredients together in a pie pan.
2. Put milk substitute in another pie pan.
3. Dip chicken in liquid, then in flour mixture and place in a baking pan.
4. Dot with margarine and bake at 425 degrees for 50-60 minutes, turning at least once.

This chicken has a very good crunchy coating.

Serves 6.

P. 14.9 C. 12.4 F. 3.4 Cal. 142.6

BOILED CHICKEN

5   pounds fowl, cut up
1   quart boiling water
1   stalk celery, sliced
1   onion, sliced
1   bay leaf
4   peppercorns
1   T. salt

1. Wash chicken and place in kettle of water.
2. Add remaining ingredients.
3. Bring to boiling point, cover and let simmer over low heat for about 2 hours, or until tender.
4. Remove from heat and let chicken cool in liquid before removing.
5. Retain liquid. Meat can be used in fricassee (see following recipe) or diced for other uses. Makes about 3 cups of diced chicken.

Serves 6.

P. 114.6 C. 3.0 F. 31.5 Cal. 779.1

CHICKEN FRICASSEE

1   boiled chicken, cut up*
4   T. milk-free margarine
5   T. rice flour
2   c. chicken stock
1   c. concentrated formula
Salt
Pepper
2   T. chopped parsley

1. Melt margarine, add flour and stir until well blended.
2. Add chicken stock and formula gradually. Stir constantly over low heat until sauce thickens. DO NOT BOIL.
3. Add salt and pepper.
4. Reheat chicken in sauce.
5. Arrange on a hot platter and sprinkle with parsley.
6. Surround with boiled rice.*

Serves 6.

P. 117.3 C. 19.9 F. 41.5 Cal. 953.7

*See index for page numbers

CREAMED CHICKEN

4   T. milk-free margarine
5   T. rice flour
1   t. salt
Pepper
1   c. chicken stock
2   c. diluted formula
2   c. diced cooked chicken
4   t. minced parsley

1. Melt margarine, stir in flour and seasonings, blend.
2. Add chicken stock and formula slowly.
3. Stir constantly over low heat until the mixture thickens. DO NOT BOIL.
4. Add chicken and parsley.
5. Reheat and serve over rice or potato nests.*

Serves 4.
P. 66.5 C. 19.7 F. 27.7 Cal. 611.7

CHICKEN IN A NEST

3   c. chicken broth
4   T. rice flour
½ t. salt
1   c. peas (if allowed)
2   c. cubed chicken, cooked

1. Make gravy with broth, flour and salt. Cook until thickened.
2. Add peas and chicken and simmer about 10 minutes.
3. Serve in potato nests,* or in a potato pie crust.*

Serves 4.
P. 68.2 C. 19.9 F. 19.3 Cal. 542.5

GOBBLERS

1   pound ground raw turkey (available ground in some supermarkets, otherwise, buy 2 drumsticks and thighs and grind, while still raw, twice in a food grinder)
1   t. salt
½ c. diced celery
3   T. minced onion
Potato flour to dip patties in
Milk-free margarine, if pan-frying

1. Carefully blend all but the flour into 4 or 5 patties.
2. Melt milk-free margarine in a frypan if you plan to broil patties.
3. Dip patties in potato flour to coat both sides.
4. Cook for 4 minutes on each side, pan-frying or broiling, until thoroughly done.

Serves 5.
P. 20.1 C. 1.1 F. 3.0 Cal. 122.0

*See index for page numbers

BROILED FISH

1   pound fish, or fish fillets
2   T. milk-free margarine or salad oil

1. Wash and fillet fish if necessary, wipe dry with cloth.
2. Brush with melted milk-free margarine or salad oil.
3. Place skin side down on well-greased broiler rack and place about 2 inches from the heat.
4. Broil until golden brown, about 10-15 minutes, until fish flakes when tried with a fork.

Serves 4 to 6.

PAN-BROILED FISH

1   pound fish or fish fillets
 ½ c. formula
1   c. crushed rice cereal or gluten-free flour

1. Wash and fillet fish if necessary.
2. Roll in formula, then in finely crushed rice cereal or gluten-free flour.
3. Melt fat in a frypan and saute fish over medium heat until brown on one side.
4. Turn with a spatula and brown the other side. Total cooking time about 10-15 minutes.

Serves 4 to 6.

BAKED FISH

1   large fish, or fish fillets to serve your family
Milk-free margarine
Salt
Pepper
Aluminum foil

1. Grease a sheet of aluminum foil that is about 3 times the size of the fish.
2. Place fish in center of foil.
3. Season fish with salt, pepper, paprika, and dot with milk-free margarine.
4. Fold foil over fish and seal tightly. Place on a cookie sheet.
5. Bake at 450 degrees for 25 minutes.

Serves 4 to 6.

COMBINATIONS AND CASSEROLES

MEAT-RICE PATTIES

1½ pound ground beef
1½ c. cooked rice
1   t. salt
2   t. tapioca flour
 ¼ c. soy base concentrate

1. Combine all ingredients in bowl.
2. Shape into patties, using ¼ cup mixture for each patty.
3. Broil for two minutes on each side. Serve hot.

Serves 6.

P. 12.2 C. 6.2 F. 8.4 Cal. 154.1

RICE AND SALMON PATTIES

¾ c. boiling water
¾ c. quick-cooking rice
1   T. milk-free margarine
2   T. potato flour
1   c. formula, diluted
1   t. minced onion
1   t. marjoram
¾ t. salt
¼ t. pepper
2   c. (1 lb. can) salmon, drained, boned, and flaked
1   c. Rice Chex, finely crushed

1. Add rice to water, cover and let stand until ready to use.
2. Prepare white sauce with flour, margarine and formula.
3. Add onion, marjoram, salt, pepper, and rice.
4. Flake salmon and add to the above mixture. If mixture is too thin to work with, add some Rice Chex crumbs to reach desired consistency.
5. Form into 8 patties and roll in crushed cereal.
6. Place on a baking sheet and bake at 450 degrees for about 30 minutes, or until brown.

Serves 4.

P. 23.0 C. 21.7 F. 8.9 Cal. 271.9

CHICKEN HASH

2   T. milk-free margarine
¼ c. chopped onion
1 ½ c. peeled, diced potatoes
2   c. diced cooked chicken
1   t. salt
½ c. chicken broth
1   T. minced parsley

1. Melt margarine in skillet.
2. Saute onions and potatoes for 10 minutes.
3 Add chicken and salt, cook 1 minute.
4. Mix in the broth and parsley, cook over low heat for 10 minutes, or until browned.

Serves 6.

P. 44.8 C. 20.5 F. 6.8 Cal. 393.8

STEAK AND POTATOES

1 ½ pounds round steak, ½ inch thick
2   T. shortening
 ¼ c. rice flour
 ¼ t. pepper
2   t. salt
1   c. home-made beef bouillon*
4   medium potatoes, pared and cut into ¼-inch slices
1   onion, thinly sliced

1. Cut steak into serving-size pieces.
2. Combine flour, salt and pepper, coat the meat with flour mixture.
3. Brown the meat slowly in shortening. This should take 20-30 minutes.
4. Add bouillon. Cover tightly and simmer (don't boil) for 30 minutes, or until almost tender. Add water if needed.
5. Place potato and onion over meat.
6. Season with salt and pepper to taste.
7. Cover tightly and cook slowly for about 35 minutes longer, or until potatoes and onions are done.

Serves 6.
P. 24.5 C. 22.1 F. 44.7 Cal. 634.2

BRISKET BANQUET

3-3 ½ pounds fresh boneless beef brisket
2   T. shortening
10   carrots, cut up
2   onions, halved
2   stalks of celery, sliced
 ¼ t. pepper
1   t. pepper
1   T. salt
6   whole cloves
6   potatoes, pared and halved

1. Place brisket in dutch oven and brown in shortening.
2. Barely cover with water and simmer, covered, for 3 to 4 hours.
3. About 50 minutes before meat is done, add potatoes.
4. Remove meat and vegetables to a hot platter.

Serves 6, with leftover meat.
1 Cup serving P. 13.0 C. 17.0 F. 19.0 Cal. 250.0

BEEF WITH RICE SOUP

1   c. home-made beef bouillon*
 ¼ c. cut up beef pieces
1   T. parsley flakes
 ¼ c. quick-cooking rice, uncooked.

*See index for page numbers.

1. Heat the bouillon and beef to boiling.
2 Add parsley and rice, stir to mix well.
3. Remove from heat and cover for five minutes.

Makes 2 servings, ¾ cup each.

P. 13.7 C. 22.0 F. 5.7 Cal. 149.8

Just because you are cooking for a restricted diet, it does not automatically follow that a lot of expense must be tolerated. Inexpensive lamb shoulder roasts make very economical meals which can be served on a restricted diet.

LAMB STEW

2   pounds lamb shoulder roast, cut up for stew
2   T. milk-free margarine
 ¼ t. granulated sugar
1   T. rice flour
2   c. lukewarm water
1   c. homemade beef bouillon*
1   medium onion studded with 1 whole clove
1   bay leaf
Pinch of thyme
 ½ t. salt
 ¼ t. pepper
12   medium-sized potatoes, pared and quartered

1. Heat margarine in Dutch oven or heavy pot.
2. Brown meat on all sides, add sugar and cook for three minutes stirring constantly.
3. Pour off fat.
4. Sprinkle meat with rice flour and cook until brown, stirring constantly.
5. Stir in water and bouillon, onion and seasonings.
6. Bring to a boil, cover and simmer for one hour.
7. Add potatoes, cover and simmer for 1 more hour and serve hot.

Makes 4 1-cup servings.

P. 50.2 C. 87.2 F. 17.7 Cal. 638.4

SHEPHERD'S PIE

2   c. ground or cooked lamb cubes
1 ½ c. lamb gravy (made with gravy recipe following)
 ½ c. peas or any allowable vegetable
2   c. cooked rice or mashed potatoes with *no milk added*
1   T. milk-free margarine

1. Grease a baking dish.
2. Spread bottom with all of rice and pour lamb mixture on top.

OR

1. Grease baking dish and fill with lamb mixture.

*See index for page numbers

2. Top with potatoes, dot with margarine.
3. Bake at 375 degrees for about 20 minutes.

Serves 4.
P. 47.6 C. 22.7 F. 70.8 Cal. 931.1

GRAVY

3 T. meat fat from roasting pan and brown juices from meat
3 T. rice or potato flour (I prefer the rice)
2 c. cold water
Salt and pepper to taste

1. Brown rice flour in roasting pan with fat and juices.
2. Slowly add water and cook over slow heat, stirring constantly, until gravy thickens and boils.
3. Season to taste.

Very good gravy—retains meat flavor.

If fats are a problem try spooning fat off juice. To remove more fat, skim surface with an ice cube. Fat will cling to the cube. This is quite time-consuming. If you plan ahead, it is easier to let the meat juices chill in the refrigerator until the fat solidifies on top and you can carefully lift it off.

Makes 2 cups.
(The following food value figures refer to a 6-tablespoon serving.)
P. 0.4 C. 3.8 F. 2.4 Cal. 38.1

LIVERICE SKILLET

¼ pound sliced bacon (if mold is not a problem) (optional)
1 pound fresh liver—beef or chicken
1 c. uncooked regular rice
3 T. snipped parsley
2 or 3 thinly sliced carrots (if allowed)
1 medium onion, thinly sliced
¼ t. salt
⅛ t. pepper
2½ c water

1. In a medium skillet, with a tight-fitting cover, fry bacon until crisp, remove, drain and crumble.
2. In bacon fat, in same skillet, saute liver until brown but still slightly pink in the center, remove from the pan.
3. Add rice, parsley, carrots, onion, salt, pepper, water and crumbled bacon to skillet. Bring to a boil.
4. Add liver. Cover and cook for 25 minutes or until rice is tender and most of the water is absorbed.

Makes 4 generous servings.
P. 22.8 C. 42.0 F. 22.4 Cal. 460.9

PORK CHOPS AND APPLES

4   pork chops
2   c. water
2   c. raw potatoes, cut up
2   c. raw apples, cut up
Salt and pepper to taste
1. Brown chops in a salted Teflon coated frypan and remove.
2. Add water and stir until all of the drippings from the bottom of the pan are mixed in. Add chops.
3. Add potatoes and cook covered for 20 minutes.
4. Add apples and simmer an additional 10 minutes.

Serves 4.
P. 30.6 C. 19.4 F. 26.1 Cal. 434.9

BRAISED HEART WITH APPLES

1   beef heart
Salt
Pepper
Potato, rice or soy flour
1   T. fat
2   T. brown sugar
2   whole cloves
2   small bay leaves
1½ c. water
2   apples, quartered and peeled
1. Wash and trim off hard parts of heart as necessary.
2. Cut in ½-inch-thick pieces.
3. Roll in seasoned flour and brown well in fat. (If you don't brown well, gravy will be gummy.)
4. Sprinkle with brown sugar, clove, and bay leaf. Add water.
5. Cover tightly and simmer about 1½ hours, until tender.
6. Add apple and continue cooking for 15 minutes.

Serves 5.
P. 10.4 C. 16.0 F. 5.3 Cal. 153.5

BEEF PORCUPINES

2   pounds ground chuck (freshly ground, if your allergies include mold)
2   c. quick-cooking rice, uncooked
½ small onion, minced
1   t. parsley flakes
⅛ t. marjoram flakes
1   t. salt
Dash of pepper
½ c. cold water

1   T. unflavored gelatin

1. Combine all ingredients except water and gelatin in a bowl.
2. Soften gelatin in cold water and pour over meat mixture.
3. Mix with hands and form into meat balls.
4. Brown in salted Teflon frypan. No fat needed.
5. Remove balls and make gravy as follows:
   2   c. hot water
   2   beef bouillon cubes, home-made bouillon* or beef tea* (two cups)
   1   T. rice flour paste (water added to flour to consistency of paste, before adding to gravy)
6. Add meatballs and simmer for 20 minutes.

Quite bland, but tasty.

Serves 4.
P. 47.7 C. 20.3 F. 29.0 Cal. 532.7

VEAL IN AN ORCHARD

4   ½-inch-thick veal chops
2   T. milk-free margarine
1   c. apple juice
 ½ c. water
 ¼ c. brown sugar
1   T. rice flour
 ½ t. allspice
2   c. raw sliced apple

1. Brown chops in fat and remove.
2. Combine remaining ingredients and add to frypan.
3. Thicken slightly and replace chops in pan, turn once.
4. Add apples and simmer covered for about 30 minutes.

Serves 4.
P. 28.1 C. 33.4 F. 49.9 Cal. 694.8

BAKED CHICKEN HASH

2   c. chicken, finely chopped
2   c. raw potatoes, finely chopped
2   T. green pepper, chopped
 ½ c. onion, finely chopped
1 ½ t. salt
 ½ c. chicken broth or water

1 Combine all of the ingredients.
2. Place in a shallow greased baking dish with a cover.
3. Bake at 350 degrees for about 1 hour, removing cover during last half hour for browning.

Serves 4.
P. 35.2 C. 27.0 F. 9.0 Cal. 333.2

BEEF STEWIE-QUE

2   pounds beef stew meat cut in 1-inch cubes
1   c. applesauce
1   t. salt
  ½ t. sweet basil
2   t. brown sugar
1   l-pound can green beans, drained
  ½ c. water
1   T. chopped onion
Shortening

1. Brown meat and onions in a little shortening.
2. Add salt, basil, brown sugar, applesauce, and water.
3. Stir until well mixed.
4. Simmer, covered, for 1 hour, then add beans.
5. Simmer covered for another hour adding water as needed.
6. Serve over rice or as a sloppy joe on Chico-san rice cakes, or rice bread* toast.

Serves 5.

P. 36.6 C. 15.6 F. 8.0 Cal. 270.4

VEGETABLES

POTATO PIECRUST

1   c. hot mashed potatoes
  ½ t. salt
1   t. cereal-free baking powder
1   t. egg substitute
2   T. water
2   T. melted shortening
Rice or potato flour (enough to make a soft dough)

1 Combine ingredients in the order given.
2. Roll mixture to about 1/8 inch thickness on a well-floured board or between 2 pieces of plastic wrap.
3. Fill with any meat filling (try *Chicken in a Nest**) and top with dabs of potatoes mashed without milk.
4. Bake in a 400-degree oven only long enough for the potatoes to brown slightly.

(Total) P. 12.0 C. 92.0 F. – Cal. 420.0

POTATO NESTS

1   2-pound bag of frozen hashed brown potatoes
Salt
Milk-free margarine to grease tins

*See index for page numbers

1. Heat potatoes in a greased frypan until thawed.
2. Salt to taste.
3. Arrange potatoes against the sides and bottom of a large deep muffin pan (or on the outside of individual custard cups and bake upside down).
4. Bake and serve hot, filled with any creamed dish. Takes about 15 minutes at 350 degrees.

It is important to grease the muffin tins VERY well before putting the potatoes in or they will stick.   Makes 6 nests.

P. 3.0 C. 21.0 F. trace Cal. 90.6

BAKED POTATO HALVES

4   medium potatoes, peeled and cut in half
½ c. water
½ c. home-made beef bouillon*
1   t. salt
¼ t. pepper
3   T. chopped parsley
2   T. milk-free margarine in small pieces
Margarine or oil to grease dish

1. Combine all ingredients in oiled or greased baking dish. and cover with aluminum foil.
2. Bake at 400 degrees for one hour, or until potatoes are tender and liquid is reduced by one-half.
3. Sprinkle with parsley and serve hot.

Serves 4.
P. 3.5 C. 21.0 F. 1.4 Cal. 104.5

SWEET BEETS

¼ c. milk-free margarine
2   T. sugar
¼ t. salt
4   c. cooked beets
¼ c. liquid if cold canned beets

1. Combine all of the above in saucepan.
2. Cook over medium heat, stirring occasionally until heated through.

Serves 6.
P. 1.3 C. 14.6 F. 3.6 Cal. 95.3

CANDIED PARSNIPS

4   large parsnips
½ c. water
¼ c. milk-free margarine, melted
¼ c. brown sugar
¼ t. salt

1. Peel and slice parsnips lengthwise.
2. Place water and parsnips in a small skillet. Salt and cover.

3. Cook for 10 minutes then add sugar and margarine, stir to coat thoroughly.
4. Continue cooking over low heat until tender and water has cooked out.
5. Turn frequently to prevent burning.

Serves 4.

P. 1.0 C. 24.0 F. 5.9 Cal. 121.5

DOUBLE BEAN PACKETS

1   1-pound can kitchen-sliced green beans, drained
1   1-pound can kitchen-sliced wax beans, drained
2   T. milk-free margarine, melted
1   t. salt
2   T. parsley flakes

1 Combine all ingredients and place in single-serving amounts in individual foil packets, using heavy-duty foil.
2. Fold foil around beans and seal tightly.
3. Bake in oven with dinner for 15-20 minutes or cook over coals for 15-20 minutes until beans are heated through.

Serves 6.

P. 1.0 C. 5.0 F. 1.8 Cal. 38.5

SQUASH BOATS

2   acorn squash, halved
6   apples, peeled and sliced
   ¾ c. brown sugar
   ½ c. milk-free margarine, melted
Dash or salt

1. Lightly salt squash halves.
2. Mix sugar and margarine and add to apples, stirring well.
3. Fill squash halves with apples (heap apples, as they cook down).
4. Place in a baking pan with small amount of water (about ½ cup) in bottom.
5. Cover tightly with aluminum foil and bake at about 350 degrees for 1 hour.
Apples retain heat, so be careful not to burn your mouth.

Serves 4.

P. 2.0 C. 77.5 F. 11.3 Cal. 398.5

FRENCH-STYLE PEAS (contains legumes)

1   c. shredded lettuce
2   10-oz. pkgs. frozen tiny green peas
4   green onions or 1/3 c. minced onions
2   T. milk-free margarine
   ¾ t. salt
   ½ t. sugar
3   T. water

1. Combine all ingredients in a saucepan.
2. Cover and cook over low heat for 25 minutes.
3. Drain any remaining liquid.
4. Taste for seasoning, add more if needed.

Serves 8.
P. 3.0 C. 9.0 F. 1.8 Cal. 59.0

ITALIAN GREEN BEAN AND POTATO SALAD

8   med. potatoes, boiled and peeled
2   c. canned green beans, drained
1   clove minced garlic
2   med. onions, chopped
1   t. salt
½   t. pepper
¼   t. oregano
1   T. sesame seeds
1   t. celery seeds
1   t. poppy seeds
½   c. cooking oil
½   c. grated Romano cheese (optional)

1. Sauté onions and garlic in a saucepan until transparent.
2. Add beans and heat thoroughly.
3. To oil, add seasonings and seeds.
4. Dice potatoes and put in a large bowl.
5. Mix oil and bean mixtures.
6. Pour over potatoes and toss gently.
7. Sprinkle individual servings with grated cheese as desired.

or

Sprinkle with grated cheese and toss again.

Serves 6.
P. 6.2 C. 37.5 F. 9.5 Cal. 260.3

MASHED POTATOES

Potatoes, sufficient for your family
Milk-free margarine
Salt
Dilute formula, if desired

1. Wash, pare, cut in pieces, and boil potatoes in water until tender.
2. Drain reserving the liquid.
3. Whip with an electric beater, adding milk-free margarine and salt to taste.

Add reserved liquid (or dilute formula) to desired consistency.

Serves number planned.

(per potato) P. 3.0 C. 21.0 F. 5.4 Cal. 138.0

RICED POTATOES

Potatoes, sufficient for your family
Parsley or paprika

1. Wash, pare, cut in pieces, and boil potatoes in water until tender. Drain.
2. Force through a ricer or coarse strainer.
3. Pile lightly in a heated dish and garnish with parsley or paprika.

Serves number planned.

(per potato) P. 3.0 C. 21.0 F. trace Cal. 90.0

FLYING W COWBOY POTATOES

(When we took a trip west and ate a chuckwagon dinner, this is how the cook at the Flying W Ranch in Colorado Springs, Colorado, cooked potatoes. I have adapted it slightly to my needs.)

4   medium potatoes
Milk-free margarine
Salt
Aluminum foil

1. Wash unpeeled potatoes.
2. Place each potato on a square of aluminum foil.
3. Add salt and a pat of milk-free margarine.
4. Wrap airtight.
5. Place in boiling water and cook until done, about an hour. They taste baked.

Serves 4.

P. 3.0 C. 21.0 F. 5.4 Cal. 138.0

BOILED RICE

2   c. cold water
1   c. converted rice
½ t. salt

1. Add rice and salt to the cold water.
2. Cover and bring to a boil.
3. Reduce heat to low and simmer for about 15 minutes.

Makes 4 ¾-c. servings.

P. 2.0 C. 22.0 F. trace Cal. 50.0

STEAMED RICE

¼ c. rice
¼ t. salt

¾ c. heated diluted formula

1. Add rice slowly to salted hot formula in the top of a small double boiler.
2. Cook for about 1 hour, until rice is tender.

Good for a sick child.

Serves 1.

P. 4.3 C. 22.4 F. 6.3 Cal. 166.4

CACKLIN' RICE

3   T. vegetable oil
½ c. minced onion
1   c. raw rice
1   t. salt
2 ½ c. hot chicken broth
3   T. parsley flakes

1. Heat oil in a skillet and saute onions for 5 minutes.
2. Stir in rice and saute until brown.
3. Add salt and broth and cook over low heat for 20 minutes, or until rice is tender and dry. Add a little water if necessary during cooking.
4. Stir in parsley.

Very good in place of potatoes. Serve with chicken.

Serves 4.

P. 4.0 C. 20.0 F. 10.0 Cal. 189.0

STUFFINGS

These stuffings can be used in place of regular bread stuffing in chicken, turkey, or pork chops.

RICE STUFFING

⅓ c. rice
½ t. salt
3   c. boiling water
½ c. diced celery
¼ c. diced onion
⅓ c. fat
5 ½ c. Rice Krispies (crushed coarsely after measuring)
2   T. minced parsley
1   T. poultry seasoning
½ t. salt
½ c. stock or water

1. Add rice to salted boiling water slowly so water continues to boil. Boil rapidly for 15-20 minutes until tender.
2. Drain in a sieve.
3. Brown celery and onion in fat.
4. Stir in rice and mix well.

5. Add parsley, seasoning and stock to crushed Rice Krispies.

6. Combine with rice and mix thoroughly.

May be baked in a covered casserole at 375 degrees for 25 minutes.

Makes 3½ cups.

(Total) P. 14.2 C. 160.7 F. 69.8 Cal. 1323.2

RICE DRESSING

¾ c. Minute Rice

2   T. oil

½ c. diced celery

2   T. chopped celery leaves

2   T. chopped onion

1   T. chopped parsley

½ t. salt

¼ t. sage

Dash of pepper

1   c. chicken broth

Chopped giblets (optional)

1. Sauté rice in oil until lightly browned, stirring constantly.

2. Add remaining dry ingredients and sauté 2-3 minutes longer.

3. Add chicken broth and mix.

4. Bring quickly to a boil over high heat.

5. Cover; remove from heat and let stand for 5 minutes.

6. Stuff bird.

Makes 1½ cups.

P. 11.5 C. 68 F. 30 Cal. 588

BOHEMIAN POTATO STUFFING

5   large potatoes

1   grated onion

1   t. caraway seeds

1   T. minced parsley

1   T. milk-free margarine, melted

1. Boil potatoes in their skins until tender.

2. Drain, peel and mash.

3. Add remaining ingredients and mix well.

Makes 4-5 cups.

(Total) P. 17.0 C. 123.0 F. 5.4 Cal. 578.0

POTATO AND CELERY STUFFING

2   onions

2   T. milk-free margarine, melted

½ c. pork sausage (contains mold)

¼ c. chopped celery leaves

5   large uncooked potatoes

   2   stalks celery
   1   t. salt
   ½ paprika
1. Dice one onion and saute in margarine until golden brown.
2. Add sausage and celery leaves and cook for 2 minutes.
3. Pare potatoes and put through a food chopper with the celery and remaining onion.
4. Add to the cooked mixture with seasoning and mix well.
5. Cook on stove, covered, for 5 minutes, then use as stuffing.

This is a very rich-flavored dressing because of the sausage; but it is quite good and excellent with turkey.

Stuffs one chicken.
(Total) P. 38.0 C. 142.0 F. 39.0 Cal. 1051.0

DESSERTS

BAKED APPLES

   6   apples
   ½ c. granulated sugar
   3   T. brown sugar

   ½ c. water
   1   T. milk-free margarine
   Cinnamon or nutmeg

1. Wash apples, core 1/3 of the way down from stem end. Arrange in a baking pan.
2. Combine sugars and water and pour over apples.
3. Dot with margarine.
4. Sprinkle with cinnamon or nutmeg. Bring syrup to a boil.
5. Cover pan and bake for about 30 minutes at 350 degrees.

Serves 6.
P. trace C. 38.0 F. 1.0 Cal. 161.0

APPLE STRUDEL

   3 ½ c. Rice Chex, slightly crushed
   2   c. sliced apples
   ½ c. brown sugar
   Dash of nutmeg
   ½ t. cinnamon
   2   T. milk-free margarine

1. Grease a covered baking dish.
2. Arrange crumbs and apples in layers.
3. Sprinkle apples with sugar, spices and dot with margarine.
4. Cover dish. Bake at 375 degrees for about 40 minutes or until apples are soft.

Serves 5.
P. 0.9 C. 35.3 F. 2.2 Cal. 165.8

10

Baking For Your Allergic Child

In order to provide a change in diet and to make sandwiches for your allergic child you will have to make bread, pancakes, muffins and the like. You will find it especially necessary for a schoolchild, because he will not be able to buy school lunches. You will also find, most likely, that the rest of your family will not eat these breads because they have a totally different flavor from the breads they are used to. The child who requires these breads however, will appreciate them.

QUICK RICE BREAD

2 c. Jolly Joan rice mix (available in health food stores)
4 t. egg replacer
4 T. water
1 c. formula, diluted
1 T. unflavored gelatin
3 T. sugar
2 T. shortening

1. Soften gelatin in formula, heat but do not boil. Let cool.
2. Add all ingredients except rice mix to the formula and combine well with electric beater.
3. Add flour until consistency of thick cake batter (still pourable).
4. Pour into a bread pan (8"x4"x2") that has been lined with foil.
5. Bake at 350 degrees for about 45 minutes. Turn out on a wire rack to cool. This bread slices best cold.

Be sure to work quickly after mixing well because this dough rises well only one time. These breads freeze well.

Makes 1 loaf (Approx. 10 slices).
(Per slice) P. 2.5 C. 29.5 F. 3.3 Cal. 158.9

RICE BREAD I (contains legumes)

2 ½ c. Fearn rice baking mix (available in health food stores)
2 t. egg replacer

  2 T. water
  1 T. unflavored gelatin
  2 T. shortening
  2 c. dilute formula or water

1. Stir gelatin into formula to soften. Heat almost to a boil, and let cool.
2. Add the egg replacer, water and shortening.
3. Beat with a mixer until well blended.
4. Add rice mix and beat until fairly smooth.
5. Pour immediately into a greased or foil-lined bread pan and bake at 350 degrees for 60 minutes.

Fearn rice baking mix contains soybean powder and carob. The bread has a more pleasing flavor than plain rice flour bread. Use only if soy is allowed on your diet.

Makes 1 loaf (Approx. 10 slices).
(Per slice) P. 1.6 C. 32.0 F. 4.0 Cal. 179.0

RICE BREAD II

  1 c. rice flour
  3 t. cereal-free baking powder
  2 T. oil
  2 T. brown sugar
  ½ t. salt
  ¾ c. water

1. Combine dry ingredients.
2. Add water and oil to dry ingredients and bake in a loaf pan at 425 degrees for 50 minutes.

Makes 1 loaf (Approx. 10 slices).
(Per slice) P. 1.2 C. 14.8 F. 2.9 Cal. 89.0

BAKING POWDER BISCUITS

  1¾ c. rice flour
  3 T. shortening
  ¼ t. salt
  3 T. formula or water
  2 t. cereal-free baking powder

1. Sift dry ingredients, cut in shortening.
2. Add liquid. Knead for 1 minute.
3. Roll to about ¾ inch thick and cut.
4. Bake at 400 degrees for about 15 minutes.

Variation:

Roll dough into a rectangle and sprinkle with brown sugar and cinnamon. Then roll as for cinnamon rolls. Slice into ½-inch pieces and place on a baking sheet. Dot with margarine and bake the same as the biscuits.

Makes about 10.
P. 2.1 C. 21.7 F. 3.8 Cal. 130.5

PEANUT BUTTER MUFFINS (contains legumes)

1   c. rice flour
4   t. cereal-free baking powder
¼ t. salt
2   T. sugar
2   T. shortening
½ c. water
3   t. old-fashioned peanut butter

1. Sift dry ingredients together.
2. Add remaining ingredients and mix well with beaters.
3. Fill greased muffin tins ¾ full.
4. Bake at 425 degrees for about 20 minutes.

Makes 6.
P. 3.7 C. 25.9 F. 8.3 Cal. 193.1

RICE CHEX MUFFINS

1   c. Rice Chex
1   c. formula
1   c. rice flour
2 ½ c. Cellu cereal-free baking powder
½ t. salt
2   T. sugar
2   t. egg replacer
4   T. water
¼ c. milk-free margarine

1. Combine Chex and formula and set aside.
2. Combine dry ingredients.
3. Add egg replacement, water, and margarine to Chex and mix well.
4. Combine with dry ingredients, stirring only until mixed.
5. Pour into greased muffin tins. Bake at 400 degrees for 25 to 30 minutes.

Makes 6.
P. 2.9 C. 31.6 F. 5.1 Cal. 183.9

RICE FLOUR MUFFINS

1   c. rice flour
2   t. cereal-free baking powder
¼ t. salt
1   t. sugar
2   T. shortening
½ c. apple juice

1. Combine dry ingredients, and cut in fat.
2. Add juice to dry ingredients and beat with mixer for two minutes.
3. Form into small patties and place in greased muffin tins.
4. Set aside to rise for 10 minutes and then bake at 400 degrees to 25 minutes.

Makes 6.
P. 4.4 C. 20.4 F. 4.7 Cal. 141.5

BLUEBERRY MUFFINS

3   T. milk-free margarine, melted
2   c. rice flour
4   t. cereal-free baking powder
 ½ c. sugar
1   t. salt
1 ½ c. fresh or frozen blueberries
2   t. egg replacer
4   T. water
1 ¼ c. milk substitute
1   t. vanilla

1. Sift dry ingredients together.
2. Mix berries with one-fourth of this mixture.
3. Beat egg replacement and add margarine, formula and vanilla. Stir into dry ingredients just enough to combine.
4. Fold in blueberries lightly.
5. Fill well-greased muffin tins ¾ full. Bake at 400 degrees for 25 minutes.

Makes 12 large muffins.
P. 2.5 C. 33.4 F. 2.4 Cal. 165.2

SOY-POTATO MUFFINS (contains legumes)

1   c. soy flour
1   c. potato starch flour
1   t. salt
2   T. cereal-free baking powder
1   T. sugar
1   T. brown sugar
 ¼ c. shortening
 ¾ to 1 c. water

1. Combine dry ingredients and mix together well. Sift.
2. Add shortening and cut in well.
3. Add water and beat with a mixer for two minutes.
4. Pour into greased muffin tins immediately, filling ¾ full.
5. Bake at 350 degrees for 25-30 minutes.

Makes 12.
P. 3.6 C. 14.7 F. 6.6 Cal. 132.6

FRESH FRUIT PIE

2   c. cut-up fresh fruit
 ½ c. fruit juice
2 ½ T. tapioca flour
 ¾ to 1 c. sugar
 ⅛ t. salt
 ½ t. vanilla
1   precooked pie crust*

*See index for page numbers.

1. Combine all but fruit in a saucepan and cook to thicken.
2. Add fruit and cook until soft.
3. Pour into pie shell after cooling for 15 minutes.
4. Refrigerate until ready to serve.

Serves 6-8.

(The following food value figures only refer to the pie filling—using apples.)

P. 2.0 C. 38.3 F. 10.8 Cal. 258.4

STRAWBERRY PIE

3   pints of fresh strawberries, washed and hulled
1   c. sugar
1   T. unflavored gelatin
     ½ c. water
Few drops of red food coloring
1   precooked pie crust*

1. Mash 1 pint of berries.
2. Add gelatin to water in saucepan to soften.
3. Add sugar and mashed berries.
4. Cook over medium heat, stirring constantly, and boil two minutes.
5. Remove from heat, stir in food coloring.
6. Cool and fold in remaining two pints of berries.
7. Pile into pie crust and chill.

Can also be served as a gelatin dessert.

Serves 6-8.

(The following food value figures only refer to the pie filling.)

P. 2.9 C. 41.7 F. 6.1 Cal. 233.3

COCONUT CRUST

3   T. milk-free margarine, melted
3 ½ oz. coconut, canned

1. Preheat oven to 300 degrees.
2. Mix ingredients and spread evenly on bottom and sides of pie tin.
3. Bake for 20 minutes or until brown.

Makes 1 crust.

P. 0.4 C. 6.2 F. 5.3 Cal. 74.1

RICE CEREAL PIE CRUST

1 ½ c. Rice Krispies or Rice Chex, finely crumbled
    ½ c. milk-free margarine, melted
    ¼ c. sugar

1. Combine ingredients.
2. Line pie pan with mixture, pressing it firmly into place.
3. Chill for 20 minutes and fill with desired filling.

Makes 1 crust.

(Total) P. 1.9 C. 83.2 F. 14.5 Cal. 470.8

*See index for page numbers.

RICE PIE CRUST

1 ¼ c. Jolly Joan rice mix (available in health food stores)
  ½ c. shortening
  4   T. cold water

1. Cut shortening into rice mix until crumbly (fine).
2. Add water.
3. Work with hands until a soft ball if formed.
4. Roll between 2 pieces of plastic wrap and place in pie pan.
5. Prick with fork to prevent buckling.
6. Bake at 400 degrees for 12-15 minutes.
7. Fill with prepared filling.

Makes 1 crust.
P. 8.6 C. 152.3 F. 100.4 Cal. 1532.5

COOKIES AND CAKES

SNICKERDOODLES

1   c. rice flour
  ¼ c. sugar
  ⅓ t. salt
1 ½ t. cereal-free baking powder
4   T. shortening
1   t. vanilla
  ¼ c. cold water
    cinnamon and sugar mixture

1. Mix dry ingredients and work the fat into them.
2. Add vanilla to cold water and then add to the dry mixture.
3. Shape dough into individual balls the size of a walnut.
4. Roll balls in cinnamon sugar mixture.
5. Press down lightly with the bottom of a glass.
6. Place on a greased cookie sheet and bake at 375 degrees for about 22 minutes.

Makes 24 cookies.
P. 0.5 C. 7.1 F. 2.3 Cal. 51.1

TAPIOCA DROPS

1   c. tapioca starch flour
  ½ c. white sugar
  ¼ t. salt
2   t. cereal-free baking powder
4   T. shortening
  ⅓ t. vanilla or almond extract
3 -4 T. cold water
  ½ c. shredded coconut or sesame coconut meal

1. Place dry ingredients into a mixing bowl and work the fat into them, much the same as for a pie dough.
2. Add water and flavoring and work dough to a soft consistency (will be sticky).
3. Add coconut and stir in.
4. Drop onto cookie sheet and flatten slightly with spoon to the same height. PLACE ABOUT TWO INCHES APART, BECAUSE THEY SPREAD.
5. Bake at 375 degrees to 10 minutes.

Makes about 2 dozen.
P. 0.1 C. 10.8 F. 3.2 Cal. 72.4

PEANUT BUTTER COOKIES (contain legumes)

½ c. old-fashioned peanut butter
½ c. milk-free margarine
½ c. white sugar
½ c. brown sugar
½ t. cereal-free baking powder
1 t. egg replacer
2 T. water

1. Combine peanut butter, margarine, both sugars, and cream until light and fluffy. (One-half cup roasted soybeans may be added if desired.)
2. Add baking powder and egg replacer and beat until smooth.
3. Drop by teaspoonfuls onto ungreased cookie sheet, about two inches apart.
4. Bake at 325 degrees for 12-15 minutes until edges are dark brown.
5. Cool on the sheet for a few minutes and remove to a plate.

Makes about 2 dozen.
P. 1.4 C. 9.4 F. 4.4 Cal. 82.8

RICE-COCONUT COOKIES

1 c. cream of rice, cooked
¼ c. sugar
⅓ t. salt
1½ t. cereal-free baking powder
¼ c. coconut
1 t. vanilla
4 T. shortening
¼ c. cold water or juice

1. Mix dry ingredients and coconut.
2. Cream into shortening.
3. Add vanilla and liquid ingredients. Mix thoroughly.
4. Shape the dough into small balls and place on greased cookie sheet.
5. Bake on top shelf of oven at 375 for 20 to 22 minutes.

Makes about 2 dozen.
P. 0.2 C. 3.9 F. 2.8 Cal. 41.6

SPICE DROP COOKIES

⅓ c. shortening
½ c. sugar
¾ c. rice flour
¼ t. cereal-free baking powder
½ t. nutmeg
½ t. cinnamon
¼ t. salt
1 T. water
1 t. vanilla

1. In a medium bowl, cream the sugar and shortening until fluffy.
2. Stir dry ingredients together and add to above mixture. Blend until smooth.
3. Beat in water and vanilla.
4. Shape dough into balls and place on an ungreased cookie sheet.
5. Flatten cookies with the bottom of a glass.
6. Bake at 375 degrees for 10 to 15 minutes or until cockies seem to have set. Remove from sheet after a few minutes and cool.

Makes about 3 dozen.
P. 0.3 C. 5.2 F. 2.1 Cal. 40.9

APPLESAUCE SPICE CAKE

2¼ c. Jolly Joan potato mix (available in health food stores)
¾ t. soda
¾ t. cloves
¾ t. cinnamon
¾ t. allspice
½ c. shortening
¾ c. brown sugar
¾ c. granulated sugar
2 t. egg replacer
½ c. applesauce
¾ c. formula or water
1 t. vanilla

1. Mix flour, spices and soda, set aside.
2. Cream shortening, sugars and egg replacer.
3. Add applesauce, formula and vanilla, mix well.
4. Gradually add dry ingredients, mixing each time until smooth.
5. Beat for 3 minutes more. Then pour immediately into greased and dusted (use rice flour) pan.
6. Bake for 20 to 30 minutes at 350 degrees.

Makes 2 layers or 24 cupcakes.
P. 0.5 C. 27.5 F. 5.0 Cal. 137.0

APPLESAUCE CAKE

½ c. milk-free margarine
1 c. sugar

    1 ½ c. applesauce
    2 ½ c. rice flour
      ½ t. cinnamon
      ½ t. cloves
    1   t. soda

1. Cream together sugar and margarine, add applesauce.
2. Sift remaining ingredients and stir into batter.
3. Mix well and pour into a greased 8-inch-square baking pan, or muffin tin.
4. Bake at 325 degrees for 40 minutes. For cupcakes, bake at 325 degrees for about 25 minutes. Cool in pan for 5 minutes and turn out on a rack.

Makes one 8-in. cake or 12 cupcakes.
P. 4.3 C. 67.8 F. 5.5 Cal. 337.9

RICE FLOUR CUPCAKES

    ⅓ c. milk-free margarine
    ⅜ c. sugar
    1   t. egg replacer
    2   T. water
      ½ t. vanilla
      ¾ c. rice flour
      ¼ t. salt
      ¾ t. soda
      ¼ c. formula
    1 ½ t. cream of tartar

1. Cream sugar and margarine thoroughly.
2. Add egg replacer and vanilla.
3. Mix and sift flour, salt, soda and cream of tartar.
4. Add dry ingredients alternately with formula. Mixture should have the consistency of cake batter.
5. Beat 3 minutes more and immediately fill paper-lined cupcake tins ¾ full.
6. Bake at 350 degrees for about 30 minutes.

Makes 12 cupcakes.
P. 0.8 C. 14.1 F. 2.6 Cal. 83.0

CARAMEL SAUCE

      ¼ c. milk-free margarine
    1   c. brown sugar
    1   t. rice flour
    1   c. cold water
    2   t. vanilla

1. Melt margarine in saucepan over medium heat.
2. Add sugar and flour which has been dissolved in water.
3. Bring slowly to the boiling point, stirring to blend.
4. Remove from heat and add vanilla.
5. Cover until ready to serve. Should mixture congeal, place over low heat.

When warm, thin to desired consistency with hot water. Beat with a spoon until smooth.

Use over baked apple desserts or over cake. Quite bland.

Makes 2 cups.

1 T. serving) P. − C. 13.3 F. 1.4 Cal. 65.8

QUICK CALAS (doughnuts)

2   c. cooked rice
3   t. egg replacer
6   T. water
 ¼ t. vanilla
 ½ t. nutmeg
 ½ c. sugar
 ½ t. salt
3   T. potato flour
3   t. cereal-free baking powder

1. Combine rice, egg replacer, vanilla, water and nutmeg.
2. Beat in a blender for two minutes, until fairly smooth. Pour into medium-sized bowl.
3. Sift dry ingredients and stir into rice mixture.
4. When thoroughly mixed, drop by spoonfuls into hot deep fat, about 360 degrees, and fry until brown, turning once.
5. Drain on absorbent paper, spinkle with confectioner's sugar, or a cinnamon-sugar mixture, or glaze with diluted Creamy Frosting, below. Serve warm or cool.

Makes 24 small doughnuts.

P. 0.2 C. 7.4 F. 0.1 Cal. 31.3

CREAMY FROSTING

6   T. rice flour
1   c. milk substitute, diluted
1   c. shortening
 ⅓ c. milk-free margarine
1   c. sugar
1 ½ t. vanilla

1. Cook flour and milk substitute until a thick paste. Cool.
2. Mix shortening and margarine and add to paste.
3. Beat very well with a mixer.
4. Add granulated sugar and beat about 5 minutes or until creamy and not grainy.
5. Add vanilla; beat to blend in well.

Has the texture of butter-cream icing. Can be refrigerated or frozen for future use.

Rewhip before using.

Makes enough to frost 24 cupcakes.

(Per cupcake) P. 0.2 C. 10.8 F. 10.7 Cal. 140.3

11

Lunches, Treats and Snacks

One of your biggest problems will be how to prepare a sack lunch for an allergic child to eat at school, on a hike, or lunch at a friend's house. There are several kinds of bread that you can make and use for sandwiches. The most puzzling question is what to use as a filling for that sandwich. Most packaged luncheon meats contain milk or hydrolized vegetable protein, and are thus unsuitable. Consider the following suggestions for sandwich fillings:

1. Chipped steak—beef cut in very thin slices by the butcher. This is a little more expensive than luncheon meat but more nourishing. Wrap in individual packets and freeze until needed. It can be pan- or oven-broiled and requires a very short cooking time.
2. Any allowed canned meat, tuna, salmon, boned bonita, etc.
3. Any leftover roast sliced thin can be frozen in small packets until needed.
4. Peanut butter and jelly if allowed, or use a peanut butter substitute.*

Now that you have a filling, how do you prepare the bread?

1. Milk-free margarine moistens the bread nicely.
2. If molds are allowed, mustard can be used.
3. Mint-flavored jelly is very good on a lamb sandwich. Try other jellies with different meats.
4. Try toasting the bread or broiling it with margarine before adding the meat.
5. Add lettuce to the sandwich.

What about the rest of the lunch? Place a milk replacement in a thermos or send small individual cans of any allowable juice. Be sure they have pop-off caps. To keep the juice cold, freeze it before placing it in the lunch. Be sure to shake it before freezing, however, or it will be very watery. Do not use a can if its top pops open in the freezer. Usually a can of frozen juice will be thawed by lunchtime just by sitting at room temperature. A can of frozen juice also helps keep the rest of the lunch cool should you include something like tuna, and have no facilities for refrigerating the lunch until time to eat.

1. Any allowable fruit can be boiled. If cooked fruit is the only kind your

*See index for page numbers.

child can eat, get a small jar to put it in or a food thermos. Use small jars of applesauce.

2. Any vegetable sticks that he likes to eat raw, such as celery, carrots, green pepper, pieces of lettuce, cabbage, cauliflower, even string beans are good raw.

Lunches needn't be a problem is you use some imagination. You will find that your child doesn't feel so left out and different from the other children if he is allowed to eat dessert, cookies, cake, ice cream, popsicles and candy. Besides, what mother doesn't like to give her child a special treat once in a while?

Without special recipes however, these treats must be completely eliminated from the allergic child's diet. Special diet cookies and desserts are somewhat more bland and gritty-tasting than normal, but they are better than nothing at all and your child will become used to them in time. You will be surprised at how relieved he is when he finds out that he doesn't have to give up ALL of the "good junk." You may even notice that you don't catch him "snitching" a food that isn't allowed on his diet as often. Here are recipes for special treats.

HONEYS

½ c. chopped roasted soybeans
½ c. honey
10 salted rice wafers

1. Combine soybeans and honey.
2. Spread on rice wafers.
3. Bake in 350 degree oven until lightly browned.

Makes 10.
P. 4.5 C. 19.6 F. 9.8 Cal. 40.6

PUFFY SQUARES CANDY

1   c. sugar
⅓ c. light brown sugar
1   c. water
½ c. salted roasted soybeans
1   t. vanilla
2   c. puffed rice

1. Make syrup from sugar and water by boiling until it reaches the soft-ball stage.
2. Add vanilla.
3. Combine soybeans and puffed cereal.
4. Pour into syrup and stir until evenly coated.
5. Turn mixture into a greased pan and cut into squares. Keeps well in an air-tight container.

Makes 20 pieces.
P. 3.6 C. 316.6 F. 10.0 Cal. 130.1

DUTCH APPLE ICE (like ice cream)

1 c. undiluted soy base
1 t. vanilla
½ t. cinnamon
½ c. white or brown sugar
1 8-oz. jar of applesauce
10 ice cubes

1. Place all ingredients except ice in a blender. Blend to combine.
2. With blender running, drop in ice cubes one at a time until crushed.
3. Pour into a bowl or small cups and freeze. This recipe can also be made as frozen pops on sticks.
4. To make like ice cream, blend in blender again after freezing and store in quart container.

This treat can also be served immediately, without freezing, like a milkshake.

Makes 3 1 cup servings.
P. 5.7 C. 71.9 F. 11.3 Cal. 402.1

LOLLIPOPS

2 c. granulated sugar
2 c. water
⅓ c. milk free margarine (optional—gives a butterscotch flavor)
1 t. vanilla extract
1 T. root beer flavoring, or any other flavoring allowed
Food coloring if desired (this recipe has a butterscotch color of its own)
40 lollipop sticks (available at cake-decorating shops, or ask your meat man for skewers)

1. Boil sugar and water slowly until it reaches the boiling point. For best results use a candy thermometer.
2. Add margarine and allow to melt.
3. Boil to 310 degrees or until threads form when dripped from spoon (hard crack stage).
4. Remove from heat and skim off top scum. Add vanilla and root beer flavoring, stir to mix well.
5. Place sticks on aluminum foil and pour candy from a spoon onto the sticks, being careful not to run candy together. Pour quickly or candy will harden in pan. If this happens, reheat until melted. These lollipops are easily removed from foil when cool.
6. Wrap individually in plastic.

Makes about 40.
P. — C. 9.6 F. 0.7 Cal. 45.0

POTATO CANDY

1 heaping T. cooked potato, whipped
3½ to 4 c. homemade powdered sugar*
1 t. vanilla
Cinnamon sugar mixture or peanut butter (legume)

*See index for page numbers.

1. Add sugar to potato in small amounts at a time and beat well.
2. Add vanilla and mix.
3. Add rest of sugar until mixture is crumbly.
4. Roll into a square between two sheets of plastic wrap until quite thin.
5. Spread with cinnamon sugar or peanut butter and roll up like a jelly roll. Squeeze to make long and slice into ½-inch slices.

This is a great recipe for the kids to help with and is very fast to make. There is no cooking involved if you use leftover potatoes with no milk added.

Makes 25 pieces.

P. – C. 32.3 F. – Cal. 125.3

COCONUT BALLS

3   T. soy base —undiluted
2   T. sugar
 ¼ t. salt
 ½ t. vanilla
1   c. moist sweetened coconut

1. Combine all ingredients except the coconut.
2. Stir in coconut.
3. Roll into tight balls and place 1 inch apart on a greased cookie sheet.
4. Bake at 350 degrees until lightly browned, about 8 minutes.

Makes 12.

P. 0.6 C. 5.7 F. 2.5 Cal. 41.7

PEANUT BUTTER FUDGE (contains legumes)

2   c. sugar
 ⅔ c. water
4   T. old-fashioned peanut butter
1   t. vanilla
Dash of salt

1. Combine sugar and water and bring to a 240 degree boil on the candy thermometer (soft ball stage).
2. Remove from heat and add the peanut butter, vanilla and salt.
3. Beat with a wooden spoon until thick and creamy.
4. Pour into an 8-inch-square pan, cool and cut into squares.

Makes 16 pieces.

P. 1.0 C. 25.6 F. 2.0 Cal. 120.0

APPLE CANDY

1½ c. water
3   c. sugar
Food coloring if desired
6   medium-sized apples

1. Make a syrup by boiling sugar and water for 5 minutes.
2. Add food coloring.
3. Wash, peel and thinly slice the apples.

4. Cook enough apples at a time to cover the surface of the syrup. Cook slowly until transparent and coated with a thick syrup.
5. If syrup becomes thick and waxy, add more water.
6. Drain apples on waxed paper, laid over a cake rack. Allow to stand uncovered for 24 hours.
7. Roll slices in granulated sugar until thinly coated.
8. Store loosely covered in a box. These have the consistency of jelly beans.

Makes 100 pieces.

(Per Piece) P. — C. 13.0 F. — Cal. 27.3

CANDY APPLES

6 apples
½ c. brown sugar
1 c. granulated sugar
½ c. maple syrup
⅛ t. cream of tartar
½ c. water
1 T. milk-free margarine
1 t. vanilla

1. Insert skewers in apples.
2. Combine all ingredients and cook to the hard brittle stage (272 degrees on candy thermometer).
3. Remove from heat and add vanilla.
4. Dip apples and cool on foil.

Makes 6.

P. — C. 87.0 F. 1.0 Cal. 288.0

KRISPIE SQUARES

1 T. unflavored gelatin
⅔ c. water
¼ c. milk-free margarine
1¼ c. sugar
3 T. light molasses or pure maple syrup
8 c. Rice Krispies

1. Soften gel in a saucepan with water.
2. Add all ingredients except Rice Krispies to the gelatin and bring the entire mixture to a boil.
3. Remove from the stove, add Rice Krispies and mix well.
4. Pour into a greased pan and allow to set overnight.

These are gummier than regular Rice Krispy squares.

Makes 20 squares.

P. 1.1 C. 23.7 F. 1.2 Cal. 107.0

MAPLE CARAMEL CRUNCH

¼ c. milk-free margarine
1   T. maple syrup
1   c. light brown sugar
4   c. Rice Chex or other allowed cereal

1. Heat margarine, syrup and sugar until boiling.
2. Cook for two minutes more.
3. While still over heat add cereal all at once, stir until thoroughly coated.
4. Spread on greased cookie sheet and cool.
5. Break into bite-sized pieces.

Makes 5 cups.
(Per ½ cup serving) P. 0.5 C. 30.6 F. 2.2 Cal. 142.8

SOYBEAN BRITTLE

2   T. shortening
½ c. boiling water
2   T. molasses
1½ cups sugar
1   c. salted roasted soybeans
1   t. baking soda

1. Melt shortening in large skillet.
2. Add water and molasses and mix well.
3. Sprinkle sugar slowly into mixture and stir until dissolved.
4. Boil until it reaches brittle stage (300 degrees on candy thermometer, or until it spins a thread when dripped from a spoon)
5. Quickly add soybeans and soda, stirring well.
6. Pour quickly onto foil, spread thin and allow to cool.
7. Break into pieces.

Makes about 20.
P. 3.4 C. 18.6 F. 11.0 Cal. 110.6

SESAME TREATS

½ c. boiling water
2   T. honey
1½ c. brown sugar
1   c. sesame seeds

1. Mix water and honey.
2. Add brown sugar and stir until dissolved.
3. Boil until reaches hard ball stage (250 degrees on candy thermometer, or test by dropping small amount into a cup of cold water.)
4. Remove from heat and add sesame seeds, mix well.
5. Drop by teaspoonsful onto foil to cool.

Makes 50 pieces.
P. 0.6 C. 17.1 F. 1.6 Cal. 81.7

12

May We Be Of Assistance?

You may find that there are times that you need answers to questions that have not been discussed in this book. Since allergies and other digestive difficulties are very individualized, it is impossible to anticipate every question you may have concerning specific foods. I have compiled a list of addresses for companies and agencies that may be able to answer any additional questions that you may have.

You most likely have already consulted with an allergist, but if not, ask your doctor to recommend an allergist in your vicinity. Once your child's diagnosis is made, there are several places you can look for help locally.

1. You allergist may have a dietitian working with him in his own office.

2. The hospital with which your doctor is affiliated may have a dietitian who could be of assistance to you.

3. Your city, county or state health department has people who can assist you at no charge. You can contact them directly or through your local school health nurse. The services that are often available are: School health nurse, visiting nurse, immunization clinic, dietitians.

4. A local university that teaches dietetics may be able to answer some of your questions.

BRANDS OF FOODS COMPATIBLE WITH RESTRICTED ALLERGY DIETS

(HFS) Health Food Store   (OSS) Oriental Specialty Store

BALANCED FOODS

Water and juice pack fruit (no salt
or sugar)

BEECH-NUT BABY FOODS

Rice Cereal (no additives)
Applesauce

Applesauce with Cherries
Applesauce with Raspberries
Peaches
Apple Juice
Apple-Grape Juice

CELLU OR
FEATHERWEIGHT (HFS)

Grainless Mix
Potato Starch
Rice Flour
Soybean Flour
Tapioca Starch
Cereal-Free Baking Powder
Featherweight Juice-Packed Fruit
   and Water-Packed fruit
Rice Wafers

CHICO SAN (HFS)

Rice Cakes
Yinnies Rice Taffy Candy (malted
   barley)
Yinnies Rice Syrup (malted barley)

DIET DELIGHT

Juice Pack Fruit

EL MOLINO MILLS (HFS)

Potato Flour
Potato Meal
Rice Flour
Soybean Flour
Caracoa (imitation chocolate)
   (carob)
Puffed Millet (gluten)
Puffed Rice
Sesame Seeds

FEARN SOY/O BRAND (HFS)

Rice Baking Mix (soybean and
   carob)

GERBER BABY FOODS

Rice Cereal (barley malt, soy)
Applesauce
Apples and Blueberries
Peaches
Plums

HAIN (HFS)

Eggless-Imitation Mayonnaise
   (gluten-free) (mold, citrus, soy)
Juices (no additives)
   Boysenberry
   Red Raspberry
Margarine (safflower—no milk)
   (soy and citric acid)
Peanut Butter Substitute
   Sesame Seed Butter
   Sesame Tahini
   Sunflower Seed Butter
Safflower Oil
Soy Oil

HEALTH VALLEY NATURAL FOODS (HFS)

Apricot Nectar with Apple Juice
Papaya with Apple Juice
Chicken Broth (no additives)

HEINZ BABY FOODS

Rice Cereal (peanut oil)
Applesauce

JOLLY JOAN (ENER-G FOODS) (HFS)

Gluten-Free Pure Rice Bran Cereal
Gluten-Free Rice Polish
Potato Mix
Rice Mix
Egg-Replacer
Baked Gluten-Free Rice Bread

NU-LIFE JUICE CONCENTRATE
(HFS) (no additives)

Apricot
Black Cherry

RALSTON PURINA

Rice Chex
Rykrisp (gluten)

TILLIE LEWIS FOODS

Juice Pack:
  Applesauce
  Apricots
  Peaches
  Pears
  Plums

MISCELLANEOUS

(OSS) Bean Threads—like spaghetti (mung bean starch)
(OSS) Dried Bean Curd Stick—like spaghetti
(OSS) Rice Sticks—like spaghetti
(OSS) Rice Vermicelli—like spaghetti
(OSS) Rice Noodles—like egg noodles (eggless)
(OSS) Rice Flake—like wide noodles
(OSS) Rice Paper—to wrap food in (edible)
       Stanfood Coconut Milk
       Newton Cream of Coconut
(HFS) Coconut Island Free-Flowing Coconut Syrup (agar agar)
       Coconut Oil (for cooking)
(OSS) Yan Chim Kee Company—Yan's Coconut Candies (corn syrup)
       Baker's Canned Flaked Coconut
(HFS) Shredded Coconut
(HFS) Midwest Arrowroot Flour
(HFS) Eden Arrowroot Flour
(OSS) String Bean Powder
(OSS) Mochiko Sweet Rice Flour
(OSS) Marukai Rice Vinegar—seasoning for salad (mold)
(HFS) Holgrain Salted Natural Rice Waferettes
(OSS) Acme Sesame Glue Rice Ball—frozen
(OSS) Summit Rice Flour—Sesame Dumpling—frozen
(HFS) Hapi Sesame Bits—rice cracker
(HFS) Ka Me Plain Rice Crunch Crackers

(HFS)   Stardust Kakoh Baby Cereal—rice cereal (oats, soy)
(HFS)   Arden Rice Cakes
         Cream of Rice Cooked Cereal
         Kellogg's Rice Krispies
(HFS)   Van Brode Low Sodium Crisp Rice (corn)
         Quaker Puffed Rice (citric acid)
         Kroger Puffed Rice
         Dae Julie Banana Chips
(OSS)   Yellow Rock Sugar—rock candy
(HFS)   Old Colony Pure Maple Sugar Candy (cut in shapes)
         Pure Maple Syrup
         Pineapple in Its Own Juice—many brands
(HFS)   Nanana—Banana Flakes (no additives)
(HFS)   Nutrafoods—Bonnie Tree Pure Vanilla Pudding and Pure Butterscotch
             Pudding (gluten free, no sugar, no additives)
         Knox Unflavored Gelatin (beef)
(HFS)
(OSS)   Agar Agar (seaweed)
         Minute Tapioca
         Minute Rice
         Tofu Soybean Curd—yogurt texture cheese (soy)
         Sexton Strained Chicken with Broth (no additives)
         All Baby Food Meats
         B & M Brick-Oven Baked Beans (no tomato or corn)
         Town Pride Canned Potato Sticks
(HFS)   Universal Foods Dry Egg Yolk (no white)
         Fleischman's Yeast (wheat-free) (corn and mold)
         Fleischman's 100% Corn Oil Margarine (soy and citric acid)
         Diet Mazola (corn, soy)
         Soft Diet Parkay (soy)
(HFS)   Willow Run Soybean Margarine
         Regular Imperial Margarine (soy)
         Diet Imperial (soy)
         PAM—Nonstick Spray for Cookware
(HFS)   Merit Apricot Honey Spread (whipped honey and apricot puree)
         Pancho Villa—Lawrey's—Ortega Taco Shells (corn and lime)
         Water Chestnuts
         Bamboo Shoots
         Morton Salt (corn free)
         Durkee's Liquid Onion Flavoring
         Molasses
         Domino Liquid Brown Sugar (use ½ as much)
         Brown Sugar
         Vita-Mite (low fat non-dairy milk) (corn)
         Schweppes Club Soda (no citrates)
         Seneca Frozen Apple Juice

(HFS)   Charisma Apple-Strawberry Juice
(HFS)   Robert's Sesame-Coconut Meal (nutty flavor)
         Most Brands Roasted:
            Soybeans
            Pumpkin Seeds (pepito nuts)
            Squash Seeds
            Sunflower Seeds
         Vita-Wheat Products (all contain soy)
            Wheat-Free Bread
            Wheat-Free Sandwich Bread
            Wheat-Free, 12 Apple Flavored Cookies
            Wheat-Free, 12 Apricot Flavored Cookies
            Wheat-Free, 12 Carob Flavored Cookies
            Wheat-Free Fruit Cake

INFORMATION AND HELP

Vita-Wheat Bakery is a family-owned business in a Detroit, Michigan suburb. It is the only bakery in the United States that bakes strictly for special diets. It has been in business since 1941 and adds new products often, at hospital request. It produces baked goods for celiac diets, food allergy diets, renal diets, diabetic diets, and salt-free/low-sodium diets. I have never met two more caring and helpful people than Jack and Richard Berry, the owners. They have a brochure containing a listing of ingredients of all their products. They will ship mail order to anywhere in the United States.
Write to:

> Vita-Wheat Baked Products, Inc.
> 1839 Hilton Road
> Ferndale, Michigan 48220

Parents of celiac children might be helped by the information sent out by the American Celiac Society. They provide new information, exchange recipes, and encourage the patients, and those who cook for them. Their address is:

> American Celiac Society
> c/o Mrs. Anita Garrow
> 45 Gifford Avenue
> Jersey City, New Jersey 07304

For general information concerning allergies, write:

> The Allergy Foundation of America
> 801 Second Avenue
> New York, New York 10017

More specific information concerning new findings, recipes, and encouragement can be obtained from:

Allergy Information Association
3 Powburn Place
Weston, Ontario, Canada M9R 2C5

Other addresses that might be of interest to you in obtaining information are:

Beechnut Baby Foods Division
605 Third Avenue
New York, New York 10016

Gerber Products Company
445 S. State Street
Fremont, Michigan 49412

Heinz Baby Food
Division of H. J. Heinz Co.
Pittsburgh, Pennsylvania 15212

Chicago Dietetic Supply, Inc. (Cellu)
405 E. Shawmut Avenue
La Grange, Illinois 60525

El Molino Mills
P. O. Box 2156
345 N. Baldwin Park Blvd.
City of Industry, California 91746

Ener-G Foods Inc. (Jolly Joan)
6901 Fox Avenue, South
Seattle, Washington 98124

Kellogg Company
Battle Creek, Michigan 49016

Ralston Purina Company
General Offices, Checkerboard Square
St. Louis, Missouri 63188

Grocery Store Products Co. (Cream of Rice)
Oakland, California 94612

Good Housekeeping Magazine
Institute/Bureau
959 Eighth Avenue
New York, New York 10019

For a small fee, they will send reprints of
articles on allergy cooking.

Appendix

ABBREVIATIONS

c. = cup   qt. = quart
T. = tablespoon   oz. = ounce
t. = teaspoon   gal. = gallon
pt. = pint

EQUIVALENTS — All measurements are level using standard measuring cups and spoons spoons

Less than 1/8 t. . . . . Dash
1 T. . . . . 3 t.
1/4 c. . . . . 4 T.
1/3 c. . . . . 5 T. + 1 t.
1/2 c. . . . . 8 T.
2/3 c. . . . . 10 T. + 2 t.
3/4 c. . . . . 12 T.
1 c. . . . . 16 T.
1 pt. . . . . 2 c. or 16 oz.
1 qt. . . . . 4 c. or 32 oz.
1 gal . . . . 4 qts. or 16 c. or 128 oz.

HALVING A RECIPE

Full Recipe . . . . Half Recipe
Dash . . . . Dash
1/4 t. . . . . Dash
1/2 t. . . . . 1/4 t.

3/4 t.	1/4 rounded teaspoon
1 t.	1/2 t.
1¼ t.	½ rounded teaspoon
1½ t.	3/4 t.
1¾ t.	3/4 t. + dash
2 t.	1 t.
2¼ t.	1 rounded teaspoon
2½ t.	1¼ t.
2¾ t.	1¼ t. rounded teaspoons
1 T.	1½ t.
1/4 c.	2 T.
1/3 c.	8 t. or 2 T. + 2 t.
1/2 c.	1/4 c.
2/3 c.	1/3 c.
3/4 c.	1/4 c. + 2 T.
1 c.	1/2 c.
1 pt.	1 c.
1 qt.	2 c. or 16 oz.
1 gal	8 c. or 64 oz.

Glossary

ALBUMIN—the chief protein component of living tissue.

ALLERGEN—any substance that causes an allergic condition.

ALLERGIC REACTIONS—any response to an allergen that is abnormal, including runny nose, itchy eyes, rash, diarrhea, vomiting, swelling, hives, difficulty breathing.

AMINO ACID—the end-product of protein metabolism which is necessary to maintain life. The body uses them to rebuild protein.

ANTIBODIES—substances produced in the blood which produce immunity.

ANTITOXIN—a substance which neutralizes the effect of a toxin (the poison released by a bacteria).

ASSIMILATE—to make part of oneself, to absorb or digest.

BIOPSY—the removal of tissue by a doctor to determine an exact diagnosis of the condition of that tissue.

CALORIES—heat units that are calculated to determine the food value of different food substances.

CARBOHYDRATE—sugar or starch.

CASSINE—a holly found in southern U.S. used as a substitute for tea. (Black drink of the Indians)

CELIAC DISEASE—a condition associated with intestinal difficulties not caused by bacteria.

CHRONIC—of long duration—not a sudden onset and cure. A condition that takes much time and patience to control but is not usually cured.

COAGULATE—to clot or thicken.

CONTACT ALLERGY—an allergic reaction caused by touching an allergen. Poison ivy is a good example.

DEHYDRATION—the extreme loss of water from body tissues.

DIARRHEA—frequent and liquid stools.

DIETITIAN—a person trained in college in the science of dietetics (the regulation of the diet to preserve health).

DUODENAL—anything concerning the first section of the small intestine—the section just below the stomach.

ELECTROLYTES—substances which can convey an electrical impulse when in solution. Body electrolytes include sodium, potassium, and chlorides, which are often lost during dehydration.

ENZYMES—the substances produced by the body to break down food so it can be absorbed in the intestines.

FAT—one of the three most important sources of calories in food.

GASTROINTESTINAL—relating to the stomach and intestines.

GLUCOSE—the simple form of sugar.

GLUTEN—a gray, sticky, nutritious substance found in many flours, which gives them a tough elastic quality when mixed with liquid.

GUARANA—dried paste made from the seeds of a Brazilian plant used to make an astringent drink.

HYPERACTIVE—sufficiently overactive to cause problems.

HYPOCHONDRIAC—one who thinks he has diseases which are not present—and is excessively and needlessly concerned over health.

HYPOSENSITIZATION ROUTINE—treatment by the doctor by using allergy injections or diet and environmental controls to lower the number of allergic reactions suffered.

IMMUNIZATION—protection against a contagious disease by injection.

ISOTONIC SOLUTION—a solution that is compatible with body tissue and one in which red blood cells can be placed without causing them to shrivel up or burst.

KHAT—African tea or Arabian tea (a stimulant narcotic).

LEVULOSE—one form of fruit sugar—a simple sugar.

MALABSORPTION SYNDROME—any poor metabolism of nutrients in the intestinal tract.

MALAISE—a feeling of being ill or unwell.

METABOLISM—the transformation of food into basic elements which can be used by the body for growth and energy.

MOLD—a downy or burry growth on the surface of organic matter caused by fungi.

MUCOUS—relating to mucus, anything that contains mucus, or has the quality of mucus.

MUCUS—a thick liquid secreted by mucous glands.

NUTRIENTS—the parts of food that help the body perform its functions correctly.

PROTEIN—a basic food substance found in all living matter.

REGULATED ALLERGY—an allergy that is under control.

SALICYLATE—the active ingredient in aspirin and many other pain-relievers.

SYMPTOMATICALLY—treatment directed toward relieving the patients' complaints rather than finding the basic cause of an illness.

THRESHOLD—the lowest level of stimulation which will produce a response (the lowest level at which you feel pain or have a slight allergic reaction).

TOXOID—a poison which has been inactivated but retains its ability to cause the formation of antibodies useful in building immunity to disease.

VILLUS (plural villi)—a stalklike growth of tissue in the mucous membrane—usually associated with absorption of food in the intestines.

Bibliography

Here is a listing of reading matter that was found most worthwhile:

Frazier, Claude A., M.D. *Coping with Food Allergy*. Quadrangle/N.Y. Times Book Co., 1974. "Food Allergies" from the *Journal of Home Economics*, Vol. 69, May 1977; p. 28.

Mosby, St. Louis. *Allergy Principles and Practice, Vols. I & II*. 1978 ed. *Nutrition and Diet Therapy Reference Dictionary, II*. Edited by Lagua, Claudio, Thiele; 1974.

Nutrition Reviews; Vol. 36, June 1978, "Breast Feeding and Management of Allergic Diseases"; p. 181. Vol. 36, Oct. 1978; "Intestinal Surface Area and Sugar Malabsorption"; p. 293.

Somekh, Emile, M.D. *Allergy and Your Child*. Harper and Row, 1974.

Speer, F., M.D. "Food Allergy: The 10 Common Offenders"; *American Family Physician*; Vol. 13, Feb. 1976; p. 106.

Taube, E. Louis, M.D. *Food Allergy and the Allergic Patient*; Revised. Charles C. Thomas, Springfield, Ill. 1978.

Index

(Recipes appear in italics under appropriate listings)